Daniel H. Grossoe

The Pastoral Care of Children

*Pre-publication
REVIEWS,
COMMENTARIES,
EVALUATIONS . . .*

"**R**everend Grossoehme's book speaks to the heart of the pastoral care of children: he provides insight into what the experience of a child is when he or she is ill and in a care setting. This is an important book for any discipline because it combines theory and application for chaplains, social workers, and others involved in the care of children. Reverend Grossoehme's respect for a child as a person shines throughout the text."

Robert Thompson, LCSW
Clinical Social Worker,
Icy River Community Care, Inc.,
Kokomo, IN

"**A** primer for ministering to our youngest parishioners, this book belongs on the desk of every parish pastor. As his namesake found God's presence in the lion's den, so does Daniel Grossoehme find the Spirit of God in the most trying of pastoral circumstances: the illness, suffering, or death of children. Mr. Grossoehme's reflective and thorough journey through the process of pediatric pastoral care provides great riches for all of us who minister to God's children."

Rev. Stuart Brooks Keith III, MDiv
Rector, Episcopal Church
of the Transfiguration,
Vail Valley, CO

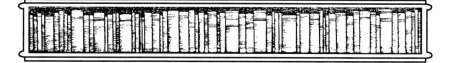

"I was thrilled to read this book. Pastoral caregivers will find it to be a gem. It has many wonderful ideas to assist them in caring for children and their loved ones. Grossoehme illustrates these ideas with many helpful examples."

Father Gerald Niklas
Clinical Pastoral Educator,
Tri-Health, Cincinnati, OH;
Author, *The Making of a Pastoral Person* and Co-Author, *Ministry to the Sick*

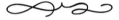

"The Pastoral Care of Children* is a book for anyone who ministers to children, desires insight into the effects of illness on children and their families, or simply cares for children. Pastors, chaplains, youth leaders, social workers, or anyone who cares about this treasure of humanity, our children, will learn and grow from reading this book. In a refreshing, conversational style, it helps unravel the mystery of children and illness. *The Pastoral Care of Children* provides practical suggestions for anyone who wants to improve his or her pastoral skills with children.

Woven throughout this book is the deep, heartfelt connection that Grossoehme has with children. It is obvious that he draws much of his inspiration for this book from the personal experience of his own compassionate ministry. This very accessible, practical book should

be in the library of anyone (not just clergy) with a heart for children and their care."

Richard D. Warger, MDiv, MNO
Executive Director,
Lutheran Chaplaincy Service,
Cleveland, OH

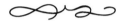

"The Pastoral Care of Children* is an excellent guide for those who are preparing to minister to children. Grossoehme addresses a wide variety of topics, including caring for children with psychiatric illnesses. Most important, he offers examples of how to talk with children in ways that respect the child. He makes a clear distinction between pastoral care and 'friendly visits.' This book shows pastors and laypeople how to offer spiritual encouragement and support appropriate to the child's age and understanding. Grossoehme understands that children speak the language of play, and in that language can speak about some scary, serious subjects. Without suggesting that his style is the only one, he offers very practical advice on how to use the tools of faith to help a child experience God's presence and God's love. As one who trains pediatric chaplains, I am delighted to have this book as a resource."

Judy Ragsdale
Associate Director of Pastoral Care,
Director of Clinical Pastoral Education,
Children's Hospital Medical Center,
Cincinnati, OH

More pre-publication
REVIEWS, COMMENTARIES, EVALUATIONS . . .

"**G**rossoehme effectively weaves together theory and practice to offer a book that is as engaging to read as it is insightful and instructive. I appreciate that his words are addressed to the ordained and lay caregiver alike, and that they are rooted in the baptismal ministry to which we all are called. Although in many ways this book is about basic pastoral care, it is also stimulating to experienced caregivers, inviting us to expand both our thinking and the faithfulness of our care. And even though Grossoehme's remarks particularly address the care of children, readers inevitably make helpful connections to the broader pastoral context. Grossoehme is refreshingly aware of children as full and complete persons who share with adults the reality of God at all times, including in illness.

Grossoehme's experience in chaplaincy and his wisdom about life, death, illness, God, and being human are gifts he carries with him into his ministry. I am grateful he has shared these gifts with the rest of us."

Rev. Canon J. A. Thompson, DMin
Christ Church Cathedral,
Indianapolis, IN

The Haworth Pastoral Press
An Imprint of The Haworth Press, Inc.

The Pastoral Care
of Children

THE HAWORTH PASTORAL PRESS
Religion and Mental Health
Harold G. Koenig, MD
Senior Editor

New, Recent, and Forthcoming Titles:

A Gospel for the Mature Years: Finding Fulfillment by Knowing and Using Your Gifts by Harold Koenig, Tracy Lamar, and Betty Lamar

Is Religion Good for Your Health? The Effects of Religion on Physical and Mental Health by Harold Koenig

Adventures in Senior Living: Learning How to Make Retirement Meaningful and Enjoyable by J. Lawrence Driskill

Dying, Grieving, Faith, and Family: A Pastoral Care Approach by George W. Bowman

The Pastoral Care of Depression: A Guidebook by Binford W. Gilbert

Understanding Clergy Misconduct in Religious Systems: Scapegoating, Family Secrets, and the Abuse of Power by Candace R. Benyei

What the Dying Teach Us: Lessons on Living by Samuel Lee Oliver

The Pastor's Family: The Challenges of Family Life and Pastoral Responsibilities by Daniel L. Langford

Somebody's Knocking at Your Door: AIDS and the African-American Church by Ronald Jeffrey Weatherford and Carole Boston Weatherford

Grief Education for Caregivers of the Elderly by Junietta Baker McCall

The Obsessive-Compulsive Disorder: Pastoral Care for the Road to Change by Robert M. Collie

The Pastoral Care of Children by David H. Grossoehme

Ways of the Desert: Becoming Holy Through Difficult Times by William F. Kraft

Caring for a Loved One with Alzheimer's Disease: A Christian Perspective by Elizabeth T. Hall

"Martha, Martha": How Christians Worry by Elaine Leong Eng

Spiritual Care for Children Living in Specialized Settings: Breathing Underwater by Michael F. Friesen

The Pastoral Care of Children

Daniel H. Grossoehme, MDiv, BCC

The Haworth Pastoral Press
An Imprint of The Haworth Press, Inc.
New York • London • Oxford

Published by

The Haworth Pastoral Press, an imprint of The Haworth Press, Inc., 10 Alice Street, Binghamton, NY 13904-1580

Cover design by Jennifer M. Gaska.

Library of Congress Cataloging-in-Publication Data

Grossoehme, Daniel H.
  The pastoral care of children/ Daniel H. Grossoehme.
    p.   cm.
  Includes bibliographical references and index.
  ISBN 0-7890-0604-9 (hc. : alk. paper). — ISBN 0-7890-0605-7 (pbk. : alk. paper).
  1. Church work with children. I. Title.
BV639.C4G74 1999
269'.22—dc21   99-34430
                                                                               CIP

For David, whose memory inspires me to care for children
and their parents as if they were my own family.

ABOUT THE AUTHOR

Reverend Daniel H. Grossoehme, BCC, is Director and Founder of the Pastoral Care program at the Children's Hospital Medical Center of Akron, Ohio. An ordained Episcopal priest, Reverend Grossoehme is a board-certified chaplain in the Association of Professional Chaplains and a member of the Executive Committee of the Assembly of Episcopal Hospitals and Chaplains. In addition to direct caregiving duties, his research interests center on how children, youth, and adults use religious language to talk with God about emotional healing and the issues they confront.

CONTENTS

Foreword

When Jesus reveals the truth of the kingdom of God to his disciples, he places a child in their midst and says, "Here. Here before you is the access to the very heart of God." Daniel Grossoehme understands what Jesus means.

This book is filled with wisdom and practical advice for anyone who cares for children, but it is mostly a book about prayer, about life, about relationships—that is—about the very heart of God.

"Groundedness," Daniel Grossoehme writes, "is very important to pastoral care. Being grounded in relationship to someone, and especially being bound to someone larger than one's own self, is the very essence of religion."

As I read through these pages, it was not long before I discovered that it is a book that is, in the most gracious way, asking me about my own groundedness. If I am going to provide pastoral care to children, then I should be ready to answer some questions for myself. Am I a person who is grounded in prayer? Can I talk about God and the love that God has for us? Can I stand before mystery? Can I name and speak the truth? Am I able to wait? How hard is it for me to be playful? How am I in the silence? Have I faced and come to terms with the reality of my own death? What does it mean to be faithful? Do I see a child as a gift from God? And can we love the child within each one of us? Where do I find blessing?

Daniel makes it clear that the gifts for pastoral care belong to us all if we are willing to enter the dying and rising that these questions require. And, as Daniel answers the questions that he has asked us, we realize that he is taking care of us, the caregivers, as well.

I will return to this book again and again because it is wondrously and carefully written, and it should belong to every person who seeks to care for children. It comes forth from Daniel's own groundedness, and through his compassion and good sense, we come to understand that Jesus is right—with the children one finds the very heart of God.

Daniel Grossoehme shows us how wide the entrance to the kingdom of heaven really is.

The Right Reverend J. Clark Grew II
Bishop of Ohio

Preface

This is a book about doing pastoral care with people under the age of eighteen. If you have picked up this book, I assume it is because you want to do this work and want to be very intentional about it. What follows is based on what children and youth have taught me in congregations, youth groups, and hospitals, about what God and their congregations mean to them. It is based on my experience, however, and comes with some of my biases and assumptions about pastoral caregivers.

I sought to make no assumptions about the ordination status of caregivers. I have used the term "pastoral caregivers" to denote any persons engaged in this work, whether clerical or lay. When I restrict something to the ordained, I have used either "priest" or "ordained minister" for clarity, but these instances are few. I also assume that the caregivers are not primarily pediatric hospital chaplains, but persons in congregations, Clinical Pastoral Education (CPE) students, and chaplains in community hospitals who do not deal with children on a daily basis.

I assume that if you want to do pastoral care of children, you are also willing to do some work by reflecting theologically on what you encounter. In perhaps no other pastoral setting do questions about God arise as when children are involved. I believe that the first time you grapple with these questions ought not to be when you are staring over a child's figure in an intensive care unit bed at distraught parents who have just asked you why God would do this to them. I have, therefore, outlined my theological thinking to date, not because it is particularly correct, or even well done, but as a model. The final set of biases arises because this book is the result of a CPE-trained Episcopal priest who does liberal theology. Read my offering, and then, as Jesus said, "Go and do thou likewise" (Luke 10:37, KJV).

Finally, this is not primarily a book about techniques. I have tried to provide a balance between praxis and theological reflection. There is no mysterious technique into which I can initiate you and turn you into someone you are not already. It is mostly a book about attitudes and relationships, both yours with children and between children and God. At the same time, there is a different approach because children have unique needs. Even though we are all former children, we forget what that experience is like, and I have sought to outline an approach that takes into account their particular needs.

I hope that you have picked out this book because you want to do pastoral care with children and youth well. When I first thought I discerned a call toward ordained ministry, I had no idea this is where I would find myself. I have resisted comments people frequently make about it taking a special person to do this work. What it takes, I have found, is someone who is willing to care an awful lot and to set aside some assumptions and fears in order to listen carefully. In spite of the pain and the tragedy I have seen, doing pastoral care with children and youth is an awesome and holy and wondrous ministry. Having children or youth talk with me about their beliefs always reminds me of Moses and the burning bush. It is a scary experience, and it is also a wonderful and sacred space. I hope that this book helps you discover this for yourself.

Daniel H. Grossoehme

Acknowledgments

I will always be deeply indebted to those who contributed to this book by forming me as priest and person: the children and youth of Christ Church (Glendale, Ohio), Holy Communion Church (Washington, DC), St. Matthew's Church (Brecksville, Ohio), and St. Peter's Church (Akron, Ohio); and those who have been patients at the Cleveland Clinic Hospital and Children's Hospital Medical Center of Akron. Several individuals have been very influential, and their thinking continues to be reflected in how I do pastoral care. These mentors include the Reverend Gerry Niklas, the Reverend Pat Persaud, the Reverend Ron Morgan, BCC, and the Reverend Dr. Ed Kryder. My colleague at Children's Hospital, Dianna VanNatter, RN, MSN, reviewed and commented on the mental health chapter. I am especially indebted to the Reverend Rod Pierce, BCC, of St. Luke's Episcopal Hospital (Houston, Texas) who read every page of the manuscript and sent it back full of questions for me to reflect on. I deeply value what you all have given to me, and this book is better because of your efforts. As much as these people have contributed to my makeup, this book and any mistakes it contains are, finally, my own responsibility.

Chapter 1

The Nature of Pastoral Care
of Children

I am sometimes apprehensive when I attend social functions for the first time. Sooner or later, I know someone will ask me what I do for a living. Even if I reply a bit vaguely, "I work in a hospital" or "I am an Episcopal priest," a follow-up question often elicits the fact that I am a pediatric hospital chaplain. This, in turn, is usually followed without a pause by a comment that takes the form of, "Oh, that must be so hard! All that suffering!" At some level, I expect those responses from the general public. What I was not prepared for was hearing similar comments from my sister and brother clergy, many of whom had been doing pastoral care substantially longer than I have.

Many persons find the prospect of working with children intimidating. In this book, I want to suggest a framework for understanding and providing pastoral care to children that is rooted in being able to express thanksgiving for children per se. Care for God's youngest children is rooted here in the act of thanksgiving for the gift of children. Jewish theology is rooted in the adoption of the Hebrews as God's chosen children; the Scriptures bear witness to their developing understanding of what that meant. Christians believe that God gave humanity the gift of a child in Christ. For them, this is the child that breaks open the cycles of life and time. Christians who give thanks for that Child can ground themselves in that thanksgiving to seek and serve Christ in the children around them today.

If that premise is the skeleton of this book, what makes the whole body function is understanding what is unique about pastoral care to children and families and how one might go about it. This is the topic of this book. Before proceeding to a discussion of the major pastoral needs of children, it is necessary to understand how children develop and the kind of thinking and spirituality they are capable of as they mature.

The reality of illness, trauma, and disease, when it occurs in children, is such that it creates an emotional tension. When people are confronted with the reality that these things can and do occur to children, they often seek to create an emotional distance from this reality. When suffering happens to children, it reminds us that no one is truly "safe," something we would like very much not to be true. These words, which make assumptions about doing pastoral care with children, also reflect a certain amount of discomfort on the part of clergypersons themselves. They may feel inadequate to the task and may not even feel called to a ministry of pastoral care. Pastoral care for children also brings up theological questions more readily—questions that have no clear and simple answers. Questions that begin "Why would God . . . ?" remind pastoral caregivers that, whatever it is that we bring to the children and families, sure and certain answers are not always part of our offering. And that causes a certain amount of discomfort and anxiety for pastoral caregivers, making it easier to talk with the parents than with the children or to avoid doing pastoral care with children entirely.

One clergyperson has related several times how in fifteen years of ordained ministry, he has never presided at the funeral of a child—and feels he is living on "borrowed time." If the pastoral care of children is a source of anxiety, it can also be a source of great joy and can be a great opportunity to learn what we really believe about God and how God operates in people's lives. The calling to be a pediatric hospital chaplain may be a unique calling, but good, solid pastoral care of children and their families can be undertaken by any person willing to put forth a bit of effort to listen to how kids talk and to what they believe about God.

The comments some people make about how emotionally difficult they find providing pastoral care to children to be serve to illustrate the confusion we feel about the suffering of children and who should tend to it. If pastoral care of children can be made to sound "different" and "special," then it becomes easier to let a specialist do it and to then permit persons based in congregations to focus their energies elsewhere. In contrast to that notion, the ordination rite for an Episcopal priest contains the instruction at the bishop's examination of the ordinand, "You are to love and serve the people among whom you work, caring alike for young and old, strong and weak . . ." (*Book of Common Prayer*, 1979). The rite leaves no ambiguity that every ordained person is to provide care to everyone, regardless of age. Yet there is no reason this care must be the sole responsibility of the ordained. The baptismal covenant, as printed in the *Book of Common Prayer* (1979), calls for all Christians to "serve Christ in all persons, loving your neighbor as yourself . . ." and to "respect the dignity of every human being" (*Book of Common Prayer*, 1979). The words from the rites of Christian initiation and ordination point in two similar directions. Everyone, including the youngest child, is deserving of pastoral care, and anyone may be the provider of that care.

WHAT IT MEANS

There is no single definition of "pastoral care" (much less pastoral care of children) to which everyone subscribes. Most people nod their heads sagely when they hear the words "pastoral care" as if everyone knows what is meant. There are, in fact, quite a few perspectives on what constitutes pastoral care; they are like each individual facet on a gemstone held up to a light that reflects differently from each facet. Each of these perspectives has a worthwhile insight into the pastoral care of children.

Clebsch and Jaekle define pastoral care as "helping acts, done by representative Christian persons, directed toward the healing, sustaining, guiding, and reconciling of troubled persons whose troubles arise in the context of ultimate meanings and concerns" (Clebsch and Jaekle, 1964, p. 4). One of the strengths of this definition is the implicit affirmation that this ministry is not limited to the ordained or licensed members of a congregation. Some persons *are* set apart for this specialized ministry, but ordination is *not* a requirement. Clergy do not have an exclusive claim to this ministry. "Representative Christian persons" is a way to affirm the uniqueness of the acts. Pastoral care is more than glad-handing people, and it is more than simply asking children at coffee hour how school is going or how their favorite sports team is doing. Simply speaking to children and youth does not necessarily communicate that they are recipients of

God's love, as adults are, in a way that sustains them through ultimate questions.

Lawrence Holst defines the role of pastoral care as "the attempt to help others, through words, acts, and relationships, to experience as fully as possible the reality of God's presence and love in their lives" (Holst, 1996, p. 46). The value of this definition is the image of balance that it brings. Pastoral care is done through the words we speak, the actions we perform, and the relationships we create and nurture. To only offer one of these, for example, to only read scriptural passages of God's healing, is not to provide pastoral care as fully as possible. The exact proportions of these three will be different depending on the caregiver's religious traditions, the age of the child, and the temperaments of the persons involved. There are times when words fail or when all words are trite: what will the pastoral caregiver have to offer then? It might be that a ritual act could speak volumes in a way that words never will. The Reformation and the fervor of the Great Awakening were valuable correctives to religious abuses or neglect going on in the mainstream church at the time. To neglect all that has been developed in the way of ritual in two thousand years of history is to neglect a huge resource, one that is particularly effective in communicating to children.

Some pastoral caregivers have the charisma to enter any situation and so immediately inspire the trust of the others present that relationships almost snap into being. Most will have to work harder, at least with some children and youth, to build and nurture their relationships. Simply being present because one has a pastoral relationship with a child, and the relationship with God that the pastor represents, is a powerful and welcome gift. The "ministry of presence," of simply being present, without need for speech or action, is not to be underestimated. Pastoral care is a matter of weaving these three strands of words, actions, and relationships together.

A very broad definition of pastoral care comes from James Fowler, who is perhaps more well known for his work of faith development. He defines pastoral care as "all the ways a community of faith, under pastoral leadership, intentionally sponsors the awakening, shaping, rectifying, healing and ongoing growth in vocation of Christian persons and community, under the presence and power of the inbreaking kingdom of God" (Fowler, 1987, p. 21). The very breadth of his definition is enough to give one pause. For our purposes, it is important to note the intentionality with which pastoral care takes place. What happens during a hospital or home visit must be based on a foundation that was built intentionally. This is how one moves beyond the greeting and begins to foster healing and growth of children who are in some way experiencing brokenness, either in body or in mind.

Awakening and shaping the growth in children's understanding of themselves as children of God, and the sense of giftedness and self-esteem that come from that, are two of the strands that I hope will clearly run through this book. Any number of people could visit a child or parents and be supportive of them, but it is the pastoral caregiver who is there to put God's words into the event. It is a special role. I have been privileged to be an invited member of a physician's discussion group about their faith and work. That invitation arose because they saw common ground with my role; as they put it, there are only two kinds of people who can show up on a family's doorstep at two o'clock in the morning and be welcomed—the child's pediatrician and pastoral caregivers. The pastoral caregiver has an awesome entrée into the lives of children and can be there to help children deal with the events of their lives in terms of their relationship with God.

Pastoral care is many things to many people. I want to refine the foregoing definitions to be more celebratory and oriented to relationships. For the purposes of this book, pastoral care is *the formation of relationships with persons of all ages that communicate (both with and without words) and bask in knowing one's self to be a child of God, so that all persons are enabled to live through their life experiences and to understand them in terms of their faith.*

WHAT IT LOOKS LIKE

Pastoral care of children is not the same as providing care to adults. Nor is pastoral care of children understood today to be mediated through their parents only. Understanding those differences is key to being able to provide care that is effective and not merely friendly. Children become sick more quickly than adults. Their bodies are smaller, and physical changes such as dehydration from vomiting occur more rapidly. Situations can become life-threatening sooner than the same event for an adult. Children also recover more quickly. It takes less time to replace their lost fluids, and they are up and well in a shorter time.

The speed at which events happen to children makes for higher levels of emotion, whether those are feelings of fear and anxiety or relief and thanksgiving. Clergy whose fears keep them from visiting children in the hospital not only avoid the feelings they expect to experience but miss the joy of seeing someone recover:

> Anthony was a six-month-old boy who had been lying on the upper bunk bed when he fell, landing headfirst on his brother, who was lying on the floor. He was brought to the emergency department with a severe head injury.

Children are so much more resilient than adults. Had Anthony been an adult male or even a teenager, his injury would likely have resulted in some form of brain damage and permanently impaired function. At six months, however, Anthony's brain is of an age that it will "rewire" itself, meaning that the neuron pathways will build detours for themselves around the damaged tissue, and Anthony has every expectation of being on par with his age-mates in virtually every way. This is not to say that the fall, hospitalization, and subsequent follow-up were not frightening for his parents. However, they found the support of prayers and pastoral visits to be a source of companionship and strength during this time.

Sickness and injury to children are emotionally difficult events because of the way in which adults, particularly parents, view children. Sometimes children are seen as a sign of hope for our future. This can be a long-term view, seeing them as carrying on our family line, or a short-term view, in which adults seek to relive their own childhoods through their children. Parents who become over-invested in their children's sporting events would be a stereotypical example of this latter category. If this is the view that adults have of their children, then any trauma or disease that threatens the children will be more threatening to adults because it is also *the adults' own sense of the future* that is threatened. Instead, when children are seen as a gift from God, the adults' own futures are no longer at stake, and an element of fear is taken away. This is not to say that an illness will not cause us anxiety and distress, but it will be because we love the child and not because we feel threatened ourselves. The focus of our emotions will be different.

One of the ways in which the early Hebrews differed from their neighbors is the way in which they understood time. Israel believed in a God who acted in history, which was seen as beginning from an initial creative event, and which was carried onward. Similar to their neighbors, they experienced life in terms of the seasons, but they saw the annual cycles as moving time forward in a linear fashion into a new future.

Israel's neighbors, by contrast, were linked to gods that controlled their agrarian lifestyle. They understood time as cyclical, moving from harvest to planting to growth and another harvest. The future was expected to be a repetition of the past and present. Any act or event that threatened the cycle threatened the entire system and was to be feared. This included hailstorms, floods, and crop damage—as well as disease and dismemberment of the workers. Fertility was valued because it increased the family's ability to participate in and perpetuate the cycle. Children's illness and death threatened the continuation of a family and its means of livelihood.

The flowing sense of time that the Hebrews conceived of mitigated this fear to the extent that they were aware there was no cycle being broken. No system's existence was threatened by the death or illness of even one of its youngest members. Children were not the product of work nor of fertility rites, but gifts freely bestowed in blessing by God. These children were understood to be without power or ability to alter their environment and, therefore, given special protection in the law along with widows. They were to be taken care of; put another way, the Hebrews were to be good stewards of their children, demonstrating thanksgiving to God by taking care of the children given to them.

These two patterns did not disappear over the centuries. Numerous children today are burdened with the expectations that they will continue the family cycle and even be things the parents were incapable of being. Listen closely at soccer and baseball games and echoes of this view of life can still be heard.

In churches that practice infant baptism, there is a symbolic action that frequently escapes notice but that reflects the theological meaning of the giftedness of a child. In this rite, it is the priest, rather than the parents, who holds the child. Water is poured, and the ritual words are spoken. Then the priest returns the infant to the family. These actions symbolically say, "Here, receive this child of God to love and nurture and raise. God gives this child into your lives—but remember that the child is always God's child."

When children are seen as gifts, it is easier to allow them to be whomever they grow into being. They are less likely to become the objects of parental projections and more likely to be valued and to learn self-esteem. Illness and death, which may threaten them, do not carry the additional burden of threatening the identity and existence of the family and its continuity. Good pastoral care prevents the need for much crisis care. In the case of children, this can be carried out by helping persons come to view children as gifts and to value their presence in community life. Some religious traditions, such as those of the Episcopal Church, have rites for the "Thanksgiving for the Birth or Adoption of a Child." Such rites may be carried out in a hospital shortly after a child is born or later in the context of the community's worship. Similar rites can be created to suit the needs of a particular congregation. Language on the part of the ordained leadership and other pastoral caregivers that reflects the giftedness of children will, in the long run, be of more help, by finding meaning in children and parenthood, than any words said in moments of tension and anxiety.

WHAT IS UNIQUE

The most fundamental way in which children are different from adults is that they use a different vocabulary to describe their experiences. They feel emotions as readily as adults but do not know the same words to describe what is going on inside them. A comment frequently heard from local clergy is, "After I get past greeting the child, I don't know what to do, so I end up visiting just the parents." What is required after the greeting is neither difficult nor mysterious but calls for a basic knowledge about how children express themselves at different ages and, on the pastoral visitor's part, the willingness to play:

Brenda was eight years old when I met her. She had been diagnosed with a brain tumor four years earlier. She had several surgeries to remove portions of the tumor. Her mother had not told her of the diagnosis nor of the upcoming surgeries until the OR team came to her room. Then she was told, "These people are going to give you something to make your head feel better." Brenda had a puppet doll named "CJ" that never left her bed. One day I noticed that the puppet wasn't there, and asked Brenda where CJ was. "She had to go away" was the reply. I asked her why CJ had to go away, and the reply, "The stuff in her head," stunned me.

It was at that point that I realized that this eight-year-old knew exactly what was going on with her disease. She simply talked about it in a different way. Over the next several months, we talked about where CJ went when she died, who she would know there (grandparents—Brenda's own grandparents having died about one year previously), about riding bicycles, and running through the grass. As long as we talked about CJ, Brenda had volumes to say and rather sophisticated ideas about what the afterlife would be like for her. One characteristic of Brenda's mother was that she wore a great deal of gold jewelry. She could be heard walking down the hallway from quite a distance. Brenda and I were in the midst of one of our deep discussions about CJ when we heard the telltale sound of her mother approaching the room. Brenda looked up and said, "We have to stop talking now—Mom cannot handle it!"

Once again, Brenda displayed astute insight. She knew what was going on inside her body; she was also aware of the dynamics between herself and her mother to the point where she knew she could not talk about her fears or her dreams. They were too much for her mother to handle emotionally.

The conversations with Brenda could never have happened if I had used her own name and inquired about what she was thinking or feeling. What made the difference was couching our conversation in terms of playfulness. Being willing to play with her made the difference. Illness is an inherently selfish experience, in that it means "self-centered." Let me hasten to state that I do not mean that in a pejorative way. We frequently talk about "the pain in my leg" or "my blood sugar level"—the focus is inward, on me. Play is what cuts through our self-centeredness. If you have ever watched toddlers or small children concentrating on playing, you understand the concept. They give play their total concentration, and they forget to be self-conscious. When playing, who the children genuinely are emerges.

The very best pastoral care will make use of this and be able to use play to reach the child. That does not mean playing board games just for the fun of it, or being friendly with the child, but using play as a tool to move beyond the child's innate self-consciousness. Pastoral caregivers will find their own unique approaches to this and will adapt them for every child. One of my hospital companions is a moose puppet. This moose wears a hospital identification badge with "Chaplain Moose" on it and sports a trademark bandanna. The moose and I often go calling together on the toddler and school-age floors because he is such a good icebreaker with these age groups. Children like to pet him and will frequently make their stuffed animal toys talk with him. Playing in this way, children feel free to express who they really are, and significant conversations have taken place that may not have except through play.

I find that inquiring about drawings a child may have around the room or offering to draw with the child can be a wonderful means of creating a pastoral conversation on the child's level. A very fine article on the use of drawing and art in pastoral care suggests ways to use drawings as a means of expression and play (Stanton, 1995). Pastoral caregivers may find it helpful to maintain a "visiting bag." This bag can be any sort of canvas tote bag with some clean paper, a box of crayons and felt-tip markers, maybe a small hand puppet or stuffed animal, a deck of cards, or other simple things that can stimulate the imagination and engage the child. Such a bag also begins to create a new identity for the pastoral caregiver. Children expect to engage in play with pastoral caregivers when they visit and expect to talk about God while they are there.

WHO MAY DO IT

Anyone may be a pastoral caregiver. I have tried to be very intentional throughout this book to avoid the use of words such as clergy and priest that clearly mean ordained persons. To the extent that people can communicate God's love and help children experience that love for themselves, they are pastoral caregivers. Nevertheless, it is usually the ordained leadership of a congregation that does the pastoral calling. Members of a congregation may expect the ordained persons to be the primary pastoral caregivers.

There are models for providing pastoral care other than the ordained person making individual calls on each person who is ill. Laypersons may also make pastoral visits, and I want to suggest that the youth of a congregation be considered as people who can be pastoral persons. There may be teenagers in a congregation who are especially articulate and responsible individuals. Consider recruiting these youth to be potential visitors. In any case, look for persons in a congregation who are emotionally healthy individuals, who seem to have good listening skills, and who display compassion for others. Such persons may be approached with an offer to talk further about doing some pastoral care on behalf of the congregation.

There are several advantages to having a teen or youth from the congregation as a pastoral caregiver. A visit from a pair of teens may be less threatening to sick children than having the minister come to visit them. Many teens have experienced baby-sitting and already have some experience relating to infants, toddlers, and young school-age children. They may be able to relate to some of the fears and other feelings more readily than adults. And they are less prone to falling into the role of acting like the sick child's parent or grandparent, which is an all-too-common pitfall of adult lay caregivers visiting children.

What these youth will need from the ordained leadership in a congregation is education and careful, ongoing support. A series of Saturday or weeknight workshops may be developed to provide education that builds on the skills they already have. Additional material on listening skills, confidentiality, and praying with children would be very helpful. Lectures that present this material are not likely to be as interesting or helpful as role-playing will be. Provide some examples of situations from your own experience, and have them role-play how they might respond. Some of the vignettes in this book might also be potential role-play material. An ordained person and other pastoral care team members can offer critiques and suggestions after each role-play. Just as with ordained caregivers, it is important that laypersons be able to focus on the child or youth and not project their own emotions onto that child.

Some thought needs to be given as to how these youth will be deployed. Who will they visit and why? Teenagers who are healthy frequently have busy lives. Their transportation needs, as well as their availability, will have to be taken into account. Their greatest value will be in visiting school-age children and peers who are sick at home for an extended period or who have lengthy hospitalizations.

Their work may supplement that of more experienced caregivers; in longer-term situations, it may even replace it. Teenagers who visit still bring with them the congregation they represent and still create community with the one who is ill. The idea of a ministry of presence, play, and community can be the overriding theme for their work.

Some formal, nationwide programs provide training and ongoing support for laypersons who wish to be pastoral caregivers. A congregation may join such a program for a fee and receive guidance on recruiting, educating, and deploying laypersons in this ministry. Or a congregation may choose to develop its own program. There are resources that provide more detailed procedures for this than is possible here (Detwiler-Zapp and Dixon, 1982). Training such persons, whether done in a formal program or with a program developed at the local level, is fundamental.

Having persons visit in teams follows the biblical precedent of Jesus sending his followers out in groups of two (Luke 10:1ff). This provides mutual support as caregivers enter the unfamiliar space of a hospital or other care center. It also provides someone with whom to process the visit afterward. Whether the lay caregivers are adults or teenagers, it is responsible to provide some means of follow-up with them. Working as part of a pastoral care team, rather than as a lone caregiver, accomplishes two things. First, it provides an opportunity to learn and grow as caregivers, by providing a mechanism to reflect on what they have done and to hear suggestions for future improvement. Second, it provides a forum for the caregivers to express and process their own feelings that have been aroused by their visit.

PASTORAL CARE AND HUMAN DEVELOPMENT

How the pastoral caregiver engages the child will change with every child. Toddlers do not play the same way a first-grade child does. After choosing to be willing to play with the child, the pastoral caregiver needs to choose with some care the words to be spoken, being informed about how humans grow and develop. Visit a fifty-five-year-old man from your congregation after cardiac bypass surgery and ask him, "How is it going with your soul?" He will almost always give you a religious, God-centered answer. Put the same question to a fifteen-year-old, and the likely response will be a blank stare. Many excellent books deal with this issue in great depth (Erikson, 1963; Fowler, 1981). What follows here is meant to be a short, practical guide to human growth and development, applied especially to pastoral care.

Consider the case of infants, generally considered to be children under the age of eighteen months:

> Pastor Cynthia complained at a local clergy meeting that she had gone to see the parents of an eight-month-old child who had been hospitalized, only to discover that the parents were not present. "There was not anything for me to do, so I left!"

Pastor Cynthia's reaction to coming into the room with only an infant is not uncommon because many people believe, at some level, that the infant is so unaware of the surroundings that significant interaction is pointless. Any parent of an infant can testify that at some level the child is capable of forming—and is seeking—trusting relationships. The world is a large, bright, cold, and sometimes frightening place filled with large, moving people. The ability to experience trust and love is critical to an infant's development. Most parents are able to provide that loving environment and experience the infant's positive response to that in return.

On a cognitive level, there is much for an infant to master. The basic human needs of food, clothing, and shelter must be attended to, and the first year is spent learning how to communicate when one or more of those needs are not being met. One anthropological reason that crying is so hard to listen to is that it is an evolutionary advantage to a helpless infant. Crying gets the attention of adults nearby and causes them to respond. Infants are also learning that they have bodies that are capable of some amazing movements.

I want to argue that the pastoral caregiver can contribute to the infant's experience of the world as a place to trust and love by the pastor's planned and intentional interaction with the infant. This is true even if, and perhaps especially when, there are no other adults in the vicinity. Pastoral care has been described as "God's love mediated" by the pastoral person to others who are hurting (Pruyser, 1976). For infants and toddlers, the pastoral caregiver is God's presence and image in the room, conveying and mediating the Divine Presence, which the infant will experience as love.

What might Pastor Cynthia have done when she visited the "empty" room when she called at the hospital? Approaching the bed with a simple, "Hi, little one!" in a gentle voice is a good beginning. Offering her little finger for the infant to grasp or offering toys are ways to interact on the infant's level. The pastor can make sure that the immediate environment around the infant is safe—physically, but also that there are toys, familiar blankets, and other comfort objects within the infant's reach. The pastoral conversation is mostly nonverbal and is more often the physical giving and taking of toys and fingers between the infant and adult. The infant does not have a word for the feelings he or she experiences, but this should not prevent the pastoral caregiver from standing in for God—being God's vicar—with that child and for seeing such an interaction as active, valid, and effective pastoral care.

Toddlers, who are generally considered to be children between eighteen months and three years old, are capable of much more interaction with the pastor. Control is a major issue at this age. This includes the beginning of controlling bodily functions as well as controlling their environment. Routines provide a sense of control because the toddlers know what to expect. Breaking routines can be upsetting to them.

The beginning of pastoral visits to toddlers may get off to a difficult start simply because the entry of the pastoral caregiver is almost certainly not a daily occurrence. The visit constitutes a break in the toddler's familiar routine. Awareness of how to respond is important. Knowing that breaking the routine is likely to be upsetting to the toddler, the pastoral caregiver can ease the situation by helping the toddler experience the pastoral caregiver as someone to be trusted. Keeping an emotionally safe distance upon entering the room, adjusting one's own height to the toddler's eye level, and speaking in a calm, soft voice are all ways to build trust. Crouching or kneeling at some distance on the floor communicates two important nonverbal messages: "I am not interested in hurting you," and "I am here to interact with you, and I will do it on your terms." Working up from there enables the toddler to accept the presence of the pastor as part of his or her world for a time, and the pastoral caregiver may then be able to interact at the toddler's level.

Toddlers have begun to experience themselves as distinct persons, different from parents and others. They can, therefore, begin to experience God as a distinct person, different from themselves. A disembodied God living in a place called "heaven" is far too abstract a concept, however. Children this age generally associate God with ministers as they are dressed for worship. An Episcopal priest vested for the Eucharist with a white alb, stole, and a poncholike chasuble is God. The person visiting on Tuesday morning is simply "Reverend John" and not God, nor even the same person as he was on Sunday. A change of context is a change of identity.

Children this age have begun to learn basic moral concepts such as right and wrong, largely through paying attention to parental reactions of approval or disapproval for every action. Parents frequently speak of the limit-pushing behaviors that toddlers engage in. Although frustrating, these behaviors are how toddlers explore their world and experience all that life has to offer at this time. They are capable not only of experiencing basic trust and love but also awe and wonder and anger. Stories from Scripture can be used to communicate God's love with toddlers. For example, stories about creation; Noah gathering the animals and God sending the flood and rainbow; Jesus eating with his disciples or gathering a crowd of children are all stories with essential truths toddlers are fully capable of grasping.

School-age children, from around four to twelve years old, live in a special world all their own. This is a time of magical thinking, when all things are possible. With their increasing verbal skills, children can express a wide range of feelings and experiences. They are generally operating at a very concrete level of thought. If an adult says God is real, then it goes without question that God is real. It is also a time of questions: if God is real, where does God live? Abstract thinking has not developed yet, and children this age often ask a series of specific questions to learn more about a new topic. For example, to say that God is "in heaven, which is above the Earth and far, far away" is to invite questions designed to elicit from the adult a verbal "map" of where God lives. Is it farther than the moon? Than Pluto? Does heaven have green grass and firm ground underfoot? In doing so, children build up a mental image of the place or person that is real to them. When they hear stories about God or God's friends, that image will be in the mind's eye as the place where the stories are enacted.

Scriptural stories are real, and believing in the miracles is especially easy. Biblical persons may be imagined as the same age as the children, and children frequently relate to them in the same way they relate to other imaginary friends—as playmates and confidantes. Faith at this stage is largely drawn from parents or other adults with whom the children have frequent contact. This is enacted physically when children attend the same church as their parents because that is where parents physically take them. The faith and values children develop largely stem from what their parents impart to them.

Magical thinking is completely normal at this stage, but it can lead to an understanding of death as a temporary condition. A sense of time is one of the last tasks of development during this period and is often not mature until the onset of adolescence. The association of death with sleep can be strong, and since people wake up each morning from sleep, and dead people look as if they are asleep, surely they will wake up from death as well. Scriptural stories about Jesus rising from the dead are taken at face value and can lead to questions about why grandparents didn't rise up and walk around after they died. Exploring this topic with children will be taken up in more detail in a later chapter.

At this stage in development, children have advanced enough that they are concerned with morality. They live by rules. Whereas rules were important for defining the limits of the toddler's world, rules enable the school-aged child to make judgments about actions. School-age children judge right and wrong based upon the consequences of their actions. Punishment, injury, or some other bad outcome will lead them to describe the act as a bad one, and perhaps one to be avoided in the future. In many instances, especially the kinds of exciting, active, risk-taking play that this age group engages in, such reasoning is often sound and helps prevent more serious injuries. It also can lead children to feel responsible for divorce, or to feel it is their fault for having an illness or injury.

Adolescence begins somewhere around the age of twelve and continues six to ten years after that. Every child develops differently, and nowhere is this more pronounced than with adolescents. Their increased abilities and sophistication with abstract and logical thinking and morality is vastly underrated by the common and reductionistic view of adolescents being hormones with feet. People sometimes comment that visiting this age group is easier than visiting younger children because of their increased verbal and thinking skills. Some people experience it as the most difficult because adolescents are often uncommunicative when they are unsure of how to relate to an individual. Understanding adolescent developmental dynamics can go a long way toward creating open relationships with teenagers.

If the work of being a child is to play, then the work of the adolescent is to take things apart. They take everything apart. Faith, values, morals—everything is open to question. Even what they formerly enjoyed doing with their parents is now reexamined and held up to a new light. That new light is most frequently the peer group. Teenagers are the most conforming people in the world, and they may temporarily shed old ideas to try on something that the group values more. At some point near the middle and end of adolescence, having taken their world apart, they begin to put it back together. What is sometimes lost in parental frustration with adolescent rebellion is that such rebellion is generally not for the sake of rebellion. A young woman ceases to be "Mary and John's daughter," creating her own identity by taking her worldview apart and becoming a person in her own right. The reassembled person often bears more than a passing resemblance to parental values—but is not merely replicating them. The root question for the teenager is, "Who am I?"

Metaphors often describe truths better than facts. The adolescent search for identity is no different from trying on various new clothes and coming out to look at one's self in the mirror. Looking at our reflection, we often ask, "Is this me?" We create our wardrobe with items that are congruent with how we see ourselves, and the other things go back to the rack. The complete ensemble rarely comes from one store. I tend to purchase my dress shirts from one particular catalog company, my ties from a local department store that carries some bright and wild patterns with fish and rainbows on them, and my shoes from another place several miles away. Adolescents do similar things with their values.

As a priest who also is available to fill in for others who are on vacation or ill, I visit a variety of congregations. In one I was treated to a complete tour by a lady who did quilting. As she showed me the current quilt in progress, she talked about how she had designed the pattern from a quilt she once saw on vacation. Other ladies were working on the quilt, and she explained that once the pattern was set, any competent quilter could come along behind her and finish the job. It struck me that this was also a good metaphor for childhood and adolescence. The patterns are set early in life by parents, but it is the work of others—of the emerging adolescent—to finish the job. Unlike a quilt, however, the pattern will very likely evolve as it moves from one end to the other.

When it comes to God, God can be either very transcendent or very immanent, depending on one's mood. God can be as easy to talk to as anyone else. Diary keeping comes readily to many teenagers, and it is easy for them to relate to the idea of journaling their prayers or thoughts about God. A pastoral caregiver, aware that adolescents are experiencing some difficulty in life, may suggest writing "letters to God" about their feelings and questions. An invitation to talk about them after one or two weeks' worth of writing would be a good follow-up. Care needs to be taken in the selection of a time and place for such follow-up, especially if the youth and pastoral caregiver are of different genders. Scriptural stories of experiences similar to what the youth are going through can also be a helpful means of assisting youth to experience God as a nearby and loving presence.

Adolescents often feel quite alone, and this can be extended to their perception of God as a far-off Being who perhaps has minimal influence or interest in their daily lives. Affirmation that this is perfectly normal can be a helpful observation to offer. If the youth are talkative, the pastoral caregiver might pursue the youth's images of God—Is God a judge seated on a high court? Is God absent from human affairs? Is God basically caring but too distant to be of any value? and so on. These images reveal much about the teenagers, and the pastoral caregiver may want to suggest other images of God that provide a "balance" to their thinking. The Psalms are replete with metaphors and similes for God and can be a resource to draw upon in such conversations.

In American culture, teenagers may have their driver's licenses and, because of that, may genuinely be able to choose whether to come to worship. This is the early expression of defining a faith that is truly theirs and not merely their parents' faith replicated. A pastoral response that permits the questions and accepts the youth's faith for where it is today will produce a more solid relationship than one that imposes the pastoral caregiver's standards upon the teenagers. Pastoral care begins by meeting the people where they are at, not where the caregiver wants them or imagines them to be.

Adolescents begin to move from making moral judgments based upon the consequences of their actions toward making judgments based upon perceived fairness to other parties. They begin to make connections between what happens to themselves and to others. One of my favorite questions to teenagers is, "How do you suppose God feels about what is happening to you?" This question cannot be used with younger children, but frequently opens an extended conversation with teenagers.

The foregoing describes normal human development. How many times have you heard or said, "I don't feel like myself today" or "I'm feeling out of sorts"? These offhand remarks nonetheless express an underlying truth: we become someone else when we are ill. Just as we speak of diseases that are in remission, when we become ill or are injured, our normal and healthy selves go into remission, and our sick selves come to the fore. Both are part of who we are as whole people, but we express different aspects of our personhood at different times.

It is normal for major experiences to cause some temporary regression in human development. Illness and injury—whether physical or emotional—are entirely capable of causing regressive changes. As we cope with the events and heal, we return at least to our accustomed level of functioning and sometimes to a bit higher level. It is worth remembering, though, that the children you visit in a hospital are not quite the same children you are accustomed to seeing in the congregation. You may need to adjust your approach to children based on the level at which you see them functioning at that time. By being aware of these changes, you can reassure parents that this "new" behavior is both normal and temporary. Seeing children regress, even a little bit, can be a source of anxiety for family members who don't understand that this is a common and normal occurrence. A good pastoral approach would assume some regression and assess early in the visit where the children are at that time.

Toddlers are learning to control their worlds, which is one reason why routines are so comforting to them; they control their world by knowing what to expect from it at any given time. Illness is unexpected and uncontrollable. Other areas in which they may have had control of life may also be thrown out of usual balance. This can range from bladder and bowel habits to disruptive sleep patterns. Eating habits may change as toddlers lose their appetites. Like infants, they may enjoy being held and rocked.

School-age children may display some behaviors usually expected of toddlers, such as demonstrations of anger and willfulness. Questions about their illness or the need to take medicines may dominate. They may feel responsible for their condition, even if it is unwarranted. They may also feel vulnerable, perhaps for the first time. They may experience the idea that, "If this happened to me once, it might happen again," and this can be a source of anxiety and fear. Such fears may be verbalized or may come out in subtle ways, such as concerns about unfinished schoolwork, being left alone, or fear of darkness. The pastoral caregiver who is aware of these changes is in a position to offer real assistance to children by helping them verbalize their fears. Bringing fears out into the light takes some of their power away.

The primary developmental task of teenagers is to form their own identities. Increasing independence from parental figures is one way they grow in this. Illness, however, may cause them to become more openly affectionate with parents and more needy of a parental presence. In the hospital, they may be reluctant for parents to leave the room. Stuffed animals may again provide a renewed sense of comfort, even for males. All of these will change as the teenagers return to their normal way of being—and some pastoral reassurance to the parents to expect this may be helpful in preventing parents' feelings of being suddenly shut out of their teenagers' lives.

> I was paged one Saturday night by a hospital nurse who told me that the mother of a four-month-old boy had asked for a chaplain to come in. The boy had been admitted for a respiratory infection and was being treated for it already. The nurse said, "I can't imagine why she wants to talk to you—the child's going to be just fine."

The pastoral caregiver's patient in this case was not the child, who was indeed going to be "just fine," as the nurse had told me. His infection was easily treated with medicine. The real patient was the mother, who told me that she was living with the boy's father and that while she wanted to get married, he was refusing. Her question was, "Is this sin? Is this infection God's punishment?"

I cite this example because it demonstrates that the illness or injury to a child, whether it is physical or emotional, affects the entire family. This book is about the pastoral care of children and youth, and they remain its focus. At the same time, quality pastoral care involves taking care of the entire family.

Pediatric hospitals have largely moved to a concept called family-centered care, which means including and involving the family in the care of the child. Family members are welcomed in pediatric hospitals and not simply tolerated, or worse, expected to be bystanders and go home after visiting hours. This concept must also be applied to pediatric pastoral care. The person with the greatest spiritual need may not be the child in the bed. The expectations and hopes that persons have for their children and themselves are frequently shaken most soundly by any illness or trauma involving a child. There are some special approaches and techniques for doing pastoral care with children, but the competent pastoral caregiver is also aware of the spiritual needs of the adults in the family constellation and provides for them as well.

Being aware of all of the families' needs, and having laid a foundation of the unique points of caring for children and youth, the next chapters will build on this foundation and explore doing pastoral care with children in more detail.

Chapter 2

Getting Beyond the Greeting

Aaron is a highly successful parish clergyperson in his mid-fifties. In spite of his success in transforming a staid, traditional congregation stereotypical for its denomination into one that is welcoming of all persons of all ages into its communal life, he expresses anxiety about visiting children. "I do not know how to have a substantive discussion with kids or youth."

Beth is the pastor of a medium-size congregation with a wide span of ages and relates that she knows she focuses more on the adults than the children. "Once I get beyond 'How are you doing?' I do not know where to go with them."

In the course of conversations with clergy whose primary ministry takes place in a congregation and who primarily do pastoral care with adults, such comments are frequently heard. Neither Aaron nor Beth is unique among pastoral caregivers for their responses. In recognizing that they feel stuck and unsure of how to proceed, they have already come to the realization that pastoral care of children and youth is different. Once over the hurdle of getting beyond the greeting, they are in a position to have some incredible discussions with children and youth. They will very likely discover that the youngest members of their congregations are frequently very willing to share their ideas about God and heaven, if only someone will show a genuine interest in hearing them.

This is not to say that getting beyond the greeting will be a simple matter. If one understands why and how it is necessary to approach children from a different perspective, then listening to them can be a grace-filled and holy experience. Understanding how pastoral care of children has its own language and style is the key to being able to minister effectively after you have said, "Hello!"

CHALLENGES FACING THE PASTORAL VISITOR

The unique style and language called for in visiting children and youth is necessary because of the developmental differences between the child and the pastoral visitor. The challenge in visiting comes from having to consciously adapt one's approach for every child. The level of adaptation necessary is also greater than how one adapts the pastoral approach taken when visiting adults. As you prepare to make a pastoral call, there are several items to pay attention to and think about.

Remember that children are very contextual. Overcoming a certain amount of stranger anxiety is to be expected when you are making a pastoral visit. When visiting an adult who is a member of a congregation, a certain level of pastoral relationship can be assumed. This is not so with children, who simply do not have the life experience to know how to respond to a pastoral visitor. Beth, the minister cited in the previous vignette, goes on to explain, "Kids seem less willing than their parents to respond to anything I have to say, so I end up visiting the adults." Since the children's experience of worship is frequently more of church school or some form of children's worship, they may rarely interact with the minister and not feel connected to that person. The nature of most worship services that children attend are still primarily geared toward adults. Although they may not be able to verbalize it, the children may not feel related to the church or its pastors. The caution here is not to assume that even children you see regularly will readily interact with you.

In addition to this distance that needs to be overcome, the pastoral caregiver may presume to have a relationship with the child simply because she or he is a member of the congregation. The child, at least at the outset, may still regard the pastoral visitor as a stranger. The pastoral caregiver teaches the child what a pastoral relationship means by modeling one. By his or her attentiveness to the child and the child's world, and through the kind of issues and conversations that take place when the pastoral person visits, the child learns that he or she has a vocabulary to talk about God and someone to do that with. Moving beyond merely greeting the child to the point of actually doing pastoral care requires more than a technique to engage conversation. It is necessary to understand how relationships are viewed and formed and to understand one's own self as a pastoral caregiver. This permits the pastor to do the work of engaging the child or youth and to move beyond mere pleasantries.

Nothing, absolutely nothing, beats having a relationship with the youth or child before there is a need to make a pastoral visit! Pastoral care is infinitely easier when the pastoral caregiver is not also meeting the child for the very first time. Of course, we all admire the pastor who is charismatic in the classical sense of that word. By charismatic, I mean those who have the ability to walk into new situations and, by their sheer presence, inspire confidence and gain the trust of the persons involved in the event. More than likely, most pastoral visitors will build trust-filled relationships over time. Obviously, then, the occasion for beginning any pastoral relationship is before an actual crisis is precipitated. Granted, this is not always possible.

Quality pastoral care of children and youth means building a relationship with them not because there is a need but because the pastoral person regards them as equal members of the congregation with intrinsic worth because they are God's children. Seeing children and youth as a gift to be enjoyed and celebrated can be a source of motivation for building relationships with God's children just for the sake of having them. Episcopal clergy have this held up in front of them in their Letter of Institution, which is read aloud at the beginning of every new ministry. They are reminded to "care alike for young and old . . ." (*Book of Common Prayer*, 1979) and they are reminded in their ordination vows to the priesthood when the bishop asks, "Will you undertake to be a faithful pastor to all whom you are called to serve, laboring together with them and with your fellow ministers to build up the family of God?" (*Book of Common Prayer*, 1979). Given that we worship and serve a God who has special concern for orphans and the young, these passages mince no words about the fact that being a pastoral caregiver means being a pastoral caregiver to every human in the congregation, from the very youngest to the most elderly. Children and youth are sometimes referred to as "the church of tomorrow," but, in fact, they are the church of today.

So, how do we begin to build those relationships with children? How do pastoral persons approach this task when they already acknowledge some discomfort and confusion? First of all, it means getting down on the children's level. In the Episcopal Church, virtually all of the Sunday worship services are Eucharists, during which the congregation comes forward to an altar rail and receives the elements, most frequently while kneeling. When I come to children under the age of twelve years or so, I enact this relationship building. I kneel down in front of them and speak directly to them as I put the bread into their hands or reach out to bless them. This reduces the intimidation factor of having a six-foot-tall, strangely dressed man tower over them. Remember, too, that young children frequently equate the clergyperson with being God, and you get some idea of what I seek to overcome. Second, this change of posture communicates to the children that this bread and these words are really intended *for* them and are not simply words said in a monotone as I pass by. The same goes for greeting persons at the end of the service. I try never to let children slip by without getting down to their level, putting my hand out to them, and greeting them. Leaning over children does not communicate interest in a relationship with them so long as you are not on the same level. Genuine eye level contact is what communicates this interest most clearly.

Opportunities to build relationships with youth abound. For clergy, acolyte training is one means of doing this. I advocate the priests doing the acolyte training themselves for several reasons. One is that whether or not the youth learn anything about ritual, I have spent some time with them and introduced myself with a bit of story about who I am and why I do what I do. I invite them to tell me about themselves. Fellowship opportunities in the life of the congregation also provide places to talk with youth. The conversations may be as light as inquiring what kind of music they listen to and how school is going in the beginning. As youth come to accept and expect a few minutes of a caring adult's time with them, they will open up more and more. Basic questions about school can develop into questions about how they make decisions concerning what they want to do after high school and what is important to them. It also sets the stage for the pastoral visit in a hospital should that ever become necessary.

Within the Judeo-Christian tradition, there is a presumption toward visiting the sick. The Episcopal rite of "Ministration to the Sick" begins with an italicized rubric that says, "In case of illness, the Minister of the Congregation is to be notified" (*Book of Common Prayer*, 1979). Presumably, the minister then acts. That action demonstrates the pastoral caregiver's awareness that the space he or she is entering is the child's room, whether it is in the home or in the hospital. Knock before entering. The child should be greeted by name, first of all. It is the child's space. Ask if it is all right for you to come in and visit. Be prepared to hear, especially from a school-age child, "No!" I am sometimes asked what to do then, to which my response is, "The child said 'No,' so it's 'no.'"

This is not to say that the pastoral visitor must turn around and leave the room, however. One might respond to the child's "no" with, "Well, how about if I just talk to your parents in the hallway, then? They can stand right here in the doorway and won't have to leave your room." The pastoral caregiver can then be in the hallway out of the child's sight and still converse with the parents. Other variations on this are possible, including suggesting that the caregiver come in and "just speak with your mom for a few minutes." However, if the child continues to say "no," then "no" it must be. Let the child know that you and God love him or her, and let the parents know you will call them later on the telephone. If you stay, in effect, you force your presence on the child, who is well-equipped to sabotage your visit by suddenly requiring parental attention, by throwing things, or by producing new symptoms that divert parental attention from your visit.

Most pastoral caregivers have invested a certain amount of time in driving to a hospital that may be located across town or in the county seat and will not be amused to have their visit so quickly turned away. Nonetheless, ending it in this fashion allows the children to have some measure of control in a situation that is largely out of their control and demonstrates respect for the children's wishes. The root message in pastoral care is that God remembers, values, and loves you, and that message has been communicated nonverbally simply by the pastoral caregiver's presence. The family knows that you care, and they will find it easier to reach out to you when the time is right.

Assuming that you are going to gain access to the room and have permission to proceed with a visit, the next question is, "Who am I going to visit?" When both the child and the parents are present, who is to be the focus? I strongly advocate that you decide on your answer to this question before you enter the room. A tension always exists when trying to answer this question. There is the shotgun approach to pastoral care, in which the pastoral visitor speaks to everyone present in the room. This approach may be dictated by time pressures (real or perceived) or by the pastoral caregiver's discomfort in playing or having a one-on-one conversation with a child. Yet there are times when a group approach to pastoral care is dictated by the circumstances. Although I firmly believe that there is pastoral value in directly interacting with children who are too young or too ill to speak with me, the focus then naturally shifts to the parents and other family members who are present. In keeping with the focus of this book, namely, that pastoral caregivers can and should be there for the child and pay primary attention to that relationship, I am going to advocate a more one-on-one approach. In general, decide who is going to be the focus of your time and stick with it.

VISITING YOUNG CHILDREN

Since you have come to visit the child, you may want to consider doing so by yourself. This means excusing the parents if they are present. Most parents find leaving the room of their sick child a difficult thing to do and may feel guilty about doing so, even if they only want to run down to the cafeteria for their own dinner. They may therefore be grateful to be given permission to leave briefly. Words such as, "How would you like to go get a cup of coffee and take a break? I'll sit here with Carlos while you are gone" or "You know, I take my role as pastor to the youth of the congregation very seriously, and I would like to talk with Daniela alone for about ten minutes. It is a gorgeous day outside; would you like to take a short walk and then come back in a bit?" will often communicate this to parents in a tactful way. It also signals to the child that you are there for him or her.

As I advocate being at the children's level when speaking to them in the congregation, it is even more important here. Sitting down—but not on their bed—is a must unless the children are up and about already. Unless you are very sure that the children know who you are, an introduction and brief statement of why you are there is in order. This last statement may be as brief as, "Mostly you see me in worship services, but during the week, much of what I do is visiting members of the congregation who are ill, so I have come to be with you for a little while." This clarifies that what is happening is a perfectly normal, though perhaps new, experience for the children. It communicates "I count in your eyes," and presumably God's, to children as members of the worship community's life.

Recall from the previous chapter that the work of being a child is to play. Play is the forum where children express their most essential being, which is who the pastor seeks to deal with. You may be able to use what is at hand in the child's room, such as a television show or video or any drawings that may have been done. Stuffed animals are always good conversation openers when they are near the child. Simple questions such as, "What are you watching?" can be developed into which character is the child's favorite, and why—which leads you to a conversation about values that highlight concerns of the child. Since characters in shows and books are real to children, it makes perfect sense to them to say, "Tell me how those characters feel when they are sick."

Sometimes there are no materials on hand to use in play with the child, and this is the point where most pastoral visitors begin to feel helpless and unsure of where to go next. They will usually change their agenda at this point and begin to visit with the adults. Being able to stay on your agenda of visiting with the child begins with some forethought. This is where you want to bring out your magic visiting bag, which contains an assortment of items. A basic list would include washable markers and scrap paper (a great way to recycle from the office); a deck of cards; a coloring book; a pair (or more) of dolls; a puppet; one or two magic tricks you know how to use. The contents of such a bag are limited only by your imagination. You may want to consider approaching individuals or a group in the congregation and ask them to sew such a bag together for you, after explaining how it is to be used. This allows people to use their skills and hobbies as a ministry and invites members to partici-pate in the ministry of visitation of the sick.

This bag becomes a recognizable part of your ministry—after some time, word will get out in the congregation that you do this—and children will expect you to have it when you come. It can be introduced with a simple, "Would you like to see what I have in here for us?" The children should be able to select what they would like to see or do. If the children are not very interactive, you may need to pick something up and begin. I often use a stuffed moose puppet, who asks the children to talk about any other stuffed ani-mals that are in the room or at home. As much fun as playing is, bear in mind that for the pastoral visitor, play is the means and not the end. What is unique about the pastoral caregiver's visit is that you are there to talk about the children's experiences and God. If the children seem inclined toward art, you might invite them to draw you a picture of what happened yesterday (or this morning, or what will happen tomorrow in surgery) or to act it out with the dolls or puppets. Or you might ask them to draw what they miss most about not being at home. The same question can be asked of stuffed animals, "What does Billy the Goat miss most about not being in the barnyard?"

Valuing children in their own right means staying with their agenda. With children, that agenda may be hidden unless you ex-plicitly bring it to light. This was brought home to me when I was visiting a young boy who recently had his appendix removed. At some point in the course of my typical conversation with children, I like to ask the question, "Can you tell me (or show me) where it hurts the most right now?" While visiting this boy, I had a vague feeling during the visit that I was missing something. He seemed full of energy for someone who just had abdominal surgery. With-out asking my usual question about where it hurt, I concluded the visit with a prayer that his tummy would feel better. I still had the feeling that I had missed something. I noticed a baseball cap in the windowsill as I was preparing to leave and decided to ask him a question about baseball just to see what might happen. His face lit up, and he lifted the sleeve of his pajamas and proudly showed off a horrible-looking bruise that he got when he made an absolutely fantastic catch but ran into the back fence! The higher than expected energy level was because he was still reliving that wonderful play from several days before. I ended up sitting down again, and we spent a delightful half hour talking about how much he liked being on a baseball team and how much the coach was a father figure for him (his own father having been killed when he was much younger). It did not require much of a leap to talk about a God who also cares for us as children and to whom we could turn for guidance and ask questions—and someone who would share our joy in making a fantastic catch! The idea that God would care about such things was a new thought for him and something he found exciting. I still believe that the part of our visit before my baseball question was "pastoral" and communicated caring to him. For me, though, the "real" visit took place only after I heard what was truly important to him.

As I started to do in that visit, many pastoral caregivers use prayer at the conclusion of the visit. I strongly advocate giving children (and adults) as much control over what happens as possible and, therefore, always ask if the child would like to pray with me or to be anointed before I leave. Again, since my theology of prayer is such that I believe God is most interested in the prayer that is in our heart (as opposed to using prayer to teach the patient what God wants or expects from us), I ask the child before I pray, "What would you like me to tell God right now?" Praying and the use of rituals with pediatric patients will be covered in more depth in a later chapter.

VISITING ADOLESCENTS

The teenager who is sick will, to some extent, be a different person from the one the pastoral visitor will know from the congregation. How different depends on many things, including the severity and kind of illness and how the child copes with illness. This calls for the pastoral caregiver to be more open to being with the teen where he or she is when beginning a visit.

Many teenagers will have stuffed animals around them on their beds. Teens should never be teased about the presence of comfort objects. Instead, use the presence of these animals as an easy way to begin conversations. One might begin simply by asking the animals' names. From there it is a simple matter to move on to, "It is nice to have Mr. Peebles with you when things are tough. I am wondering if you can tell me about the most difficult thing you are thinking about right now."

If you have ever been hospitalized or been seriously ill, you might build rapport with a youth who doesn't know you well by telling what that experience was like for you. Even a teen who knows you from the congregation probably hasn't seen this side of you before. This expression of empathy creates some shared experience between you and the teen. It will build trust in the relationship and help make you seem more approachable. Teenagers are primarily going about the work of determining their own identities. With teens, conversations that accept them and treat them as maturing individuals will go a long way toward building rapport and respect. Much of the basic material about visiting with children holds with adolescents: acknowledge the room as theirs; excuse parents, at least sometimes; adapt your posture to be on their level.

Teenagers are frequently very open to questions and very often are reflective thinkers. They are often very open to dreaming with you about God's response to them. One of my favorite questions to pose is, "What do you suppose God is thinking right now about what has happened to you?" Youth are frequent journalers, although adolescent women tend to call them diaries. The pastoral caregiver can inquire if a journal of some sort is kept and suggest that they write down what this experience has been like for them. One can suggest that many people feel better after doing this. Questions about what is happening to them or about God might come up, and one could invite the youth to discuss these questions after they are feeling better.

VISITING WITH THE PARENTS

There will certainly be times when pastoral caregivers will want to specifically visit with the parents. This will be more familiar territory because it more resembles the traditional visiting of adults they are accustomed to doing. Simply because a child is involved, the emotional level is apt to run a bit higher. Some issues peculiar to visiting adults who are parents need to be highlighted.

There is a saying in chaplaincy circles, "Do not just do something—sit there!" One of the most frequent complaints that parents have made to me about being visited by the clergy from their congregation is that the pastor's own level of discomfort was so high that the pastor simply was not emotionally or spiritually present to them. Simply because many clergy do not frequently visit pediatric patients in a hospital, some level of unease is natural. Discomfort often takes the form of finding an activity, frequently a religious activity such as prayer or a rite, that the priest knows well and can at least put the priest on more familiar ground. In being so busy "doing" they miss the opportunity to simply be present in front of the burning bush and stand quietly on holy ground. Sometimes that discomfort manifests itself in trite sayings that are meant to console or explain God's unfathomable actions. Words have tremendous power, and a healthy respect for that is helpful for pastoral visitors. Sometimes it is better for pastoral caregivers to speak no words at all. Instead, they can listen, allowing the mystery that is the other person's suffering to unfold with the telling of his or her story. When pastoral caregivers rush in with answers, situations such as the following have occurred:

> Ellen was the mother of a four-year-old boy diagnosed shortly after birth with a chromosomal abnormality. She was at that time just beginning to attend a church, having been away from religion for twenty-five years. Around her son's third birthday, he was diagnosed with a form of cancer. When Ellen, still reeling from the impact of this new diagnosis, told her pastor, the response was, "Well, I would not rule out the possibility that God is cursing this child!"

One of the things that I have gained from pediatric chaplaincy is a stronger appreciation for the mysterious. I can represent God in this place and can remind people of God, but I cannot supply all of the answers. I have heard and seen too many events to pretend that I have any special insight into the mind of God. Words that wound are very easy to speak and, I believe, are more easily spoken when one loses a sense of humility and gains a desire to control everything through being certain of all the answers. In my experience, most people do not have pastors such as Ellen's, yet similar comments are made by pastoral visitors who mean well but say wounding words. Comments about God's will after the death of a child or the loss of a pregnancy and suggestions that there are or can be other children fall into this category. Parents who have heard such comments relate that it would have been better for the minister to just sit there in silence with them and soak up the tension than to speak words, however well-meant, that are remembered and hurtful months and years later.

One of the dimensions of visiting a child in the hospital is that the likelihood of meeting multiple family members is higher than when visiting an adult. All visitors there have their own feelings and issues, some of which are related to the problem at hand and some of which are not. Listening to the concerns of various people in situations such as this is like processing sounds from multiple radios set to different stations! How the pastoral visitor handles this is largely a matter of personal style. A card-carrying introvert, I deal with fifty-two family members in the emergency department in much the same way I deal with the parents, speaking more or less privately to one or two people here, and then this small group over there, and so on around the room. Other ministers prefer addressing multiple family members as a whole and engaging them as a community to pray or cry or support one another as a group. Almost any approach is appropriate, and sometimes the nature of the crisis may dictate the pastoral style offered. Generally, the pastoral caregiver may expect to encounter large groups of people more often when visiting children than when visiting adults.

> Francis, age eleven, was recently diagnosed with diabetes. The parents were frightened of the changes in lifestyle and eating that the family might have to make. In conversations with the chaplain, they spoke of resenting having to reshape their lives around their son's disease.

Parents may have very strong feelings that need some pastoral attention even though they are not the patients. These parents are an example. Anger or resentment may build, if not vented, which covertly sabotages medical maintenance of the diabetes; Francis could return to the hospital, quite ill. In cases of this sort, I find it helpful to wonder aloud about the child's illness or injury. Will there be any long-term implications? How will the family cope with changes in diet or the daily management of insulin injections? Francis's diabetes and his parents' concerns and feelings certainly have some pastoral implications. Pastoral caregivers in congregations arc in an excellent position to help such families cope with long-term issues because they have longer-term relationships. Such pastoral interventions need not be formal or intense but can be as simple as, "I am wondering how you are all doing having to monitor Francis's blood sugar and diet."

It is generally a good idea to inquire whether the parents feel their questions have been adequately answered by their physicians. If not, encourage them to make a list of questions for their doctor; most physicians appreciate such an effort. It demonstrates concern for the child's care and respect for the physician's time. Some families cope by asking *lots* of questions—using information as the primary coping skill. This can certainly be an appropriate coping skill and is a necessary part of a healthy grieving process. An excessive use of this coping mechanism can also be a way to avoid dealing with the spiritual and emotional dimensions of illness. Intuition plays a part in understanding the family dynamics.

Coping with information generally occurs very early in the disease process—while waiting for a diagnosis and the period shortly thereafter. The condition must be named and understood before it can be dealt with, just as the demons were cast out of the Gerasene only after their name, "Legion," was known (Mark 5:1-20). At some point, the pastor will sense that the time is right to invite the child and perhaps the family into a deeper discussion. This might take the form of, "You certainly have a great deal of information about Wilm's tumor. I am wondering how you and God are doing with this right now." It is a mistake to force people to confront an emotion before they are ready for it, and difficult diagnoses do require a long adjustment period. Some persons will be so devastated by the medical news that they will be in shock and emotionally numb. Questions about meaning or God may have to wait for hours or days before they can be asked. During the initial stage, when shock is common, an abiding presence with the child and family is the best approach. Many pastoral caregivers seek to ask these questions long before the child or the family is ready to answer them. A discomfort in abiding with people in pain pushes pastoral caregivers to leap into naming the demon, saying a prayer that defines them as the dispenser of spiritual remedies, and pronouncing that the road to healing has begun. The invitation to reflect on the experience on a deeper level will only be accepted by a child or youth after the pastoral caregivers have demonstrated that they are an ongoing presence that can be trusted. After being with the child when he or she is given information about his or her condition and helping the child express himself or herself, then the invitation to talk more deeply can certainly be made; whether or not it is pursued remains up to the child or parent.

It is important to remember that each family member will react differently. A stereotypical dad who is "in control" and attending to details is not necessarily one who is unfeeling, unaffected, or unhurt. A gentle, "How about you?" to quiet family members may bring out some different issues about the illness or injury that need to be dealt with. Silence does not always mean agreement.

FAMILY SATISFACTION WITH PASTORAL VISITS

Viewing children and their families as clients to be satisfied is not an especially helpful image for pastoral care. On the other hand, most pastoral caregivers would like to do a good job and be thought of as good pastors of their congregations. For clergy who serve churches with a congregational polity (where they serve at the pleasure of a lay governing body), their jobs may literally depend upon the positive feelings of those for whom they care. An interesting study was published that looked at how clergy who visited children with cancer were perceived by both the children and the parents (Spilka, Spangler, and Nelson, 1983).

Clergy who made insensitive comments about the children or their conditions were one of the primary causes of people's upset. These included comments such as that made by Ellen's pastor in the previous vignette. Suggesting that it is God's will for a child to die—whether or not the pastoral caregiver believes this to be true—or that people should pray for an outcome they are not ready for are other examples of this category. Poor communication, especially about the reason for the visit, also made for bad feelings. Parents and children report being able to sense when clergy were visiting them out of a sense of duty. "Why am I here?" would be a question to pose to one's self in the hallway. If the only answer is "I am the pastor and I am supposed to visit," then it may be worth spending some time reflecting on how one sees pastoral ministry. If the pastoral visitor is devoid of any sense of mediating the Divine presence or of helping people connect or reconnect with their God, this will be communicated to the children.

Pastoral caregivers might begin their initial greeting not only with their name but with the reason for the visit. This sets up clear communication about who they are and why they are here. This can be as simple as "Hi, Tanesha! I wanted to come and talk with you for a little while."

If children and parents were able to pick up on feelings that the clergy were visiting them out of a sense of duty, they seemed even more able to pick up on feelings of discomfort. Looking at one's watch frequently during a visit and failing to physically enter the room are two examples of this. Pastoral relationships cannot be built when the child is in a bed and the pastoral caregiver is leaning against the doorway.

Most pastoral caregivers are probably unaware of the little habits that communicate their feelings. A technique used in Clinical Pastoral Education is that of a joint visit in which two students make a pastoral visit together, but one person is responsible for being aware of the interpersonal skills of the other and for providing feedback in a private place after the visit. An observer is in a good position to notice the odd little habits that communicate discomfort, such as abrupt changes of topic. Pastoral visitors might make use of these learning methods during the course of their visiting and invite a trusted member of the congregation, another pastor, or a hospital chaplain to accompany them and provide feedback afterward. Issues about confidentiality should be discussed with the observer beforehand. A brief word of explanation to the child or family might be in order as well so that they do not wonder "who else knows" or what the observer might say afterward.

"Doing nothing" was the most common complaint made by children or their parents in this study. On the one hand, this suggests that there were differing expectations about what happens when a clergyperson visits. It is not hard to envision a pastoral caregiver who puts a high value on a ministry of presence, a child who cannot figure out why this person is just sitting there making small talk with Mom, and a parent who wants a prayer but is afraid to ask. On the other hand, many people reported being very happy simply because the pastor came to them. Many persons view their clergy as busy people and do not want to be an additional pastoral burden to them. When a clergyperson did make time to visit, it made a meaningful impact upon these persons, and they were grateful.

Interestingly, this study concluded that the clergy generally considered their pastoral efforts to be far more effective than the children and parents whom they visited. A significant portion of the complaints made about clergy visits can be seen as a conflict between different (and unspoken) expectations. Pastoral caregivers who take advantage of a variety of opportunities to talk about what they do and the meaning behind their care, who ask what people would like from them, are more likely to find themselves meeting others' expectations. Newsletters and youth or adult education hours provide forums to present what pastoral care looks like within one's religious tradition and within this particular worshiping community. Constructive feedback from parishioners can be obtained after a significant event by inquiring, "for the sake of those I care for in the future," about what the parishioners found to be the most and least helpful.

PASTORAL IDENTITY

One of the assumptions I made when beginning to write this book was that any pastoral caregiver willing to pick up this book and work through it is willing to put some effort into doing pastoral care well. If the pastor has been intentional about the purpose of a pastoral visit, who the intended recipient of pastoral care is going to be, and has succeeded in gaining entrance to the child's room, there remains one final issue. Understanding what my role is before I enter a room sets the context for my pastoral care. How I see myself influences how I interact with people and what I do during a visit.

Without such self-awareness, pastoral caregivers tend to offer the same care to every child without considering what each child's unique needs and abilities are. Some children may be too sick to talk or draw; others may need to vent their anger or grief. Some ways of presenting myself are more inviting to children than others. Being aware of how I present myself allows me to choose, within the limits of my personality, how to be most open and inviting to others. Without paying attention to such issues, pastoral caregivers and the children they visit may easily become confused over what each person expects.

I had a mentor who used to claim that there were at least six persons present in every pastoral encounter. They are the person whom you see, the person I know myself to be, the person I project to you, the person whom I see, the person you know yourself to be, and, finally, the person whom you feel you project to me during the visit. With every additional body in the room, the number of persons increases by the power of three. It is not hard to see how confusion over who I am can arise. To avoid confusion and unmet expectations, it is important for pastoral visitors to have a sense of who they are as pastoral caregivers. This does not need to be firm and fixed, nor does it mean that one slips into a pastoral role as easily as one puts on a jacket.

Children and youth frequently have no experience of their clergy outside of worship or youth group. They may not have any experience with any other pastoral caregiver from the congregation. It is up to the pastoral caregiver to define what the role is and to give shape to what that looks like. Having a clear sense of one's pastoral identity, or the various identities that one uses, is a helpful way to be clear to yourself and to the children in your care who you are and what "pastoral care" looks like. Having a self-understanding of what it means to you to be a pastoral caregiver, and the ways in which you intend to communicate God's word and presence, increases the likelihood of effective pastoral care.

Each of us who provide pastoral care move in and out of several pastoral identities. They are formed by our personalities, our sense of what it means to be a minister, the types of interactions we are comfortable with, and the age and condition of the child or youth we are visiting. Generally speaking, some pastoral identities are more comfortable for us than others and some are more or less helpful to the children we care for.

Being a child's *Playmate* can be a way to build a nonthreatening relationship with a child and to be intentional about spending time with him or her. This is a quiet, companionable role that centers on some playful activity. Open-ended questions can be posed by the pastoral caregiver while drawing or shuffling cards, and the child or youth can gently be engaged on an emotional or religious level. Somewhat similar are the *Community Builders,* who visit because they believe that their very presence in the room creates a worshiping community and ends the isolation from the congregation that the child may experience. At the least, they serve to remind the child of his or her link to a congregation. Community Builders often are also Playmates.

Playmates can also adopt the role of *Clown.* The Clown's visit is always entertaining and children often laugh and have a good time. The Clown may tell jokes, perform a magic trick, or simply tell stories. This in turn makes the pastoral Clown feel good about what has been done and increases the likelihood of these kinds of visits in the future. While the Clown can certainly be a Community Builder, it can be difficult to shift to a deeper emotional level during the visit. Since children readily accept this form of adult visitation, they may quickly come to expect it of all pastoral visits, which locks the pastoral visitor into a single dominant role. This is by no means meant to denigrate clown ministries, which do bring joy to children. It is difficult, though, if not impossible, to be both a clown and the children's pastoral caregiver. If you have a clown ministry, decide beforehand which one role you want to have with these children.

There are times when what a child really needs above all else is someone to listen. Pastoral visitors may come to see themselves as *giant Ears for God.* There is little need for them to say anything beyond minimal prompts; the child or youth is generally someone who is very verbal and articulate and has a great deal to say. In some respects this is similar to the doing nothing role that parents complained about in a previous example. This misperception of the pastoral caregiver as one who does nothing is the danger of adopting this particular identity. The crucial difference is that, in its best form, being an Ear is an active role, not a passive one. This is not simply sitting there nodding from time to time but using active listening skills. The pastoral caregiver reflects back to the child what was heard and makes use of prompts and other minimal encouragements to enable the child to tell the story as fully as possible.

It is sometimes necessary to confront a child or youth. Much of contemporary pastoral care is based on simple, nonjudgmental listening. This is often summarized by talking about meeting people where they are. This approach works well much of the time, but one may find that there are some youth with whom this approach does not work. This is frequently the case when substance abuse, behaviors related to conduct disorders, and even normal adolescent rebellion is involved. Rather than meeting the youth where they are, it may be necessary to stand firmly where one's beliefs are and call the youth to a place where they are not. This is the work of the *Prophet.* God's prophets have always stood where the people were not and called to them with the *Lord's* words.

A final pastoral image to consider is that of the pastor as the *theologian in residence* in a congregation (DeGruchy, 1986). While at first blush this may appear to be limited to the ordained person, or too academic, it need not be so. Laypersons do have the opportunities for some theological training, both formal and informal. In the case of pastoral theology, it would be well for the church to recover a sense of all persons being able to do "practical theology" because all persons can reflect upon their experiences in terms of their beliefs and values.

When this image has been presented for discussion it has often been met with reactions of skepticism and outright dismissal. This may stem from a reluctance to claim the title of theologian because of its association with academic centers rather than the experiences of daily living. Despite this criticism, the image is still a useful one, for it serves as a reminder that all persons who do pastoral care speak God's words by their words or deeds, and so do theology. A second way in which this image is useful is that it is accessible to persons of a wide variety of traditions. To see myself primarily as a priest may lead me to emphasize the sacramental elements of pastoral care; to see myself primarily as someone whose religious tradition arose out of the Reformation may lead me to ignore the sacramental elements in favor of Scripture reading or simply conversing (DeGruchy, 1986). The image of the pastoral caregiver as one who can listen and interpret the human experience of brokenness in light of one's beliefs is to be the theologian in residence in a worshiping community.

The images of pastoral identity described here are only a tiny portion of how pastoral caregivers might imagine their ministry. None are necessarily right or wrong, although some may be more helpful to the pastoral visitor or to the child or family than others. Their value is not in labeling or categorizing ("I am God's Ear today and so all I intend to do is to listen"). Nor should they be used to provide an excuse to reduce one's self to less than the fullness of one's calling ("I am just God's Ear"). The value of these identities, and other related ones, is in helping a person be more focused and intentional about visiting and its purpose. A clear image of who one is will be reflected in what happens when you enter.

Chapter 3

Pastoral Issues
in Acute Care Settings

When people imagine doing pastoral care with children, I find that acute situations are usually what they picture in their mind's eye. In part this really is because children tend to have acute problems. It is also because these are highly emotional events that bring up ultimate questions for which pastoral caregivers often have no simple answers. Acute issues require children and youth to confront, possibly for the first time, their fondly held notion, "It cannot happen to me." Henri Nouwen suggests that the suffering that many persons experience is caused not by an event itself but by the faulty assumptions that they have made about their lives. These assumptions can include the ideas that one who believes in a good God ought not to be afraid or confused or lonely (Nouwen, 1972).

The practical issues described in the previous chapters may all be brought into play in an acute setting, whether this takes place in an emergency room, surgical waiting area, or some other acute care area. There are some emotions that pastoral caregivers will more likely encounter here and encounter at a greater depth than in more routine areas, and they are the focus of this chapter. These include fear, anger, and guilt. Each of these can lead to feeling isolated from God and from family members.

FEAR

Events can happen suddenly with children. This happens when they are playing; it also happens to their bodies when they get sick, when they have an accident, or are struck. In a moment, life can change very rapidly. That very suddenness creates anxiety: what is wrong? Is it permanent? Each person experiences those feelings differently, and that can lead to a sense of isolation.

Trauma: Fearing the Worst

> My trauma pager beeped to announce the impending arrival of an ambulance carrying a small boy from an automobile accident. As the squad's doors opened, the boy's mother stepped out first and came into the emergency department running next to the stretcher. She looked frantic with worry and close to tears. Part of my job is to take her to another area and be with her there.

The separation of the child from the parent is one of the emotional difficulties of doing pastoral care in acute situations. It is helpful to understand the basis of the fear. It is almost always present, even if it is not voiced explicitly. Having an understanding of the more primal fear underneath the words and emotions helps shape and influence the practical aspects of pastoral care. What cannot be seen is more easily feared. Many parents have expressed how difficult it is to know that their child is hurting and to feel helpless because they cannot fix it. Some voice the fear, "What if they take her somewhere and will not let me go with her?" Without the visual connection to their child, they fear losing the physical connection as well. No matter how gracefully and graciously I do it, one of the effects of trauma, which I help enact, is the separation of a family. It is part of my job that I find difficult to do. I understand the staff's desire to focus solely on the patient and their fear of having a parent suddenly faint and become a patient as well. Meanwhile, we sit apart from the child.

Trauma brings with it, at least temporarily, an uncertain outcome. That uncertainty over the immediate future tears a gap in the fabric of family relationships. For a period of time, not only are children and parents separated physically, but they all usually fear a more permanent separation. Human beings are not isolated individuals, but rather are connected and related to one another by birth, adoption, and marriage. Those threads of connection are threatened most when an injury or illness is so acute that the child must be brought to a hospital emergency department or an intensive care unit.

Uncertainty over the outcome manifests itself in different ways. Since children are physically separated from their parents, they may be fearing the complete loss of a living relationship. If the child is seriously injured, family members may be wondering if they are still so-and-so's parent or sister or brother. To some extent, any trauma has the capacity to shake the foundation of one's identity. And so I find it important to be as concrete as possible in the beginning. The first questions are clustered around answering, "Who are you? Who am I? And why are we here?" When I meet a family in the emergency department, one of my first questions is, "What is your child's name?" Oddly, many parents have to stop and think for a moment before replying. Their world has been so profoundly shaken that they have lost their sense of groundedness and relationship.

Beginning a visit in the emergency department with such a simple question as "What is your child's name?", accomplishes two things. First, it is far more respectful to talk about the child by name rather than "your daughter" or "your son" or "your kiddo." Second, simple questions such as this help persons who have lost their sense of groundedness to recover it. By being asked concrete questions, they are given something simple to focus upon, and they usually regain a sense of control over themselves and over the seeming chaos around them.

Groundedness is very important to pastoral care. Being grounded in relationship to someone, and especially of being bound to someone larger than one's own self, is the very essence of religion. The etymology of "religion" is the root *ligio*, meaning "to tie or to bind," and the prefix *re-*, meaning again. Religion is what binds us and ties us together with one another and with God. Relationships are reciprocal. Parents experience over anxiety over the one they belong to; there is also a concern for who belongs to them. Helping people reforge those connections is the work of religion and its representatives who are pastoral caregivers.

Benno, a pastor with ten years' experience, was called to the hospital after a seven-year-old boy, Steven, was involved in an accident at home. Benno sat with the family in the hospital's emergency department waiting room and also with Steven in his curtained-off area. In reflecting later on his two-hour experience, Benno commented that sitting around with people waiting for news and bringing coffee to them was not his idea of pastoral ministry, especially in a hospital. He left very frustrated by this experience.

Acute situations involving children cause fear. On the surface this fear is the loss of a child's usual ability to play or to interact with family members, and sometimes it is even fear of death. The actions that one does or words that one speaks are less important than the relationship that is present. Benno's frustration arose when his sense of pastoral identity did not fit with the experience of sitting with the patient and family and bringing them coffee. Perhaps nowhere else is the simple ministry of presence called for than in acute or emergent situations. The ability to keep silent, to hold a hand, and to wait with a child can say more about God's concern for children than any words the pastoral caregiver might speak. In sitting quietly, one makes visible the bond that exists between the child and the One to whom they are bound: God.

Simply by being present in silence in the midst of chaos allows an opportunity for God's Spirit to work. It provides space for people to give voice to their fears and hopes. It is a creative time. Consider the author of a book who begins with an idea, then moves toward words on a page, then chapters one by one, and finally, to the birth of a new and whole creation. The word author has the same roots as the word authority. To have authority is to use one's self in such a way that new life comes into being. We grant authority to those who have given something new to our lives. Silence is a sign of authority in the most literal, creative meaning of that word.

Surgery: Fearing the Unknown

The majority of surgeries that children undergo are relatively brief and simple. Tonsillectomies or putting tubes in the ears are such short and routine procedures that there is a temptation to dismiss them as too insignificant for a pastoral care visit. The procedure may take only thirty minutes and allow the family to be home in time for lunch, but from the parents' perspective, it will be a very long half hour until the surgeon appears and says, "Everything went fine." Parents have often commented, "When it is your child, there is no such thing as a 'minor' surgery."

To consider the surgery from a child's perspective, reflect on the following example:

> The anesthesiologist stepped up to the bed where eight-year-old Benjamin was waiting, along with his parents and the pastor, for surgery to begin. After the doctor introduced himself to the parents, the mother turned to Benjamin and said, "This is the doctor who is going to put you to sleep." Benjamin's eyes grew wide and then he began to sob uncontrollably.

The mother's remark seems innocent enough, but Benjamin had heard the expression "put to sleep" used as a euphemism for what a veterinarian (a kind of doctor!) does to kill injured pets. Knowing something inside of him needed fixing and finding a strange doctor standing in front of him, Benjamin's reaction is almost predictable. Fear is the primary pastoral issue that children having surgery experience. It can include fear of the unknown; fear of separation from the parents; fear of the staff; fear of not waking up; or fear of feeling the cutting of the knife.

Many pediatric hospitals have sophisticated programs, usually staffed by Child Life specialists, that address the normal fears of children. Some allow for tours of the operating rooms and walk the children through every step in the process from the time their names are called until they wake up in the recovery room. The tours involve medical play, which desensitizes the children to the new equipment and how it will be used on their bodies. Such experiences help children (and adults) cope with having surgery. In most community- or adult-centered hospitals, children probably have not had this preoperative experience, and their fears, even for a short and simple procedure, may well be quite high.

Fear is a way we build walls around us to protect ourselves; it keeps us from willingly going into threatening situations. If children have their walls built up because of the fears they have, it may be very difficult for pastoral caregivers to communicate or represent God to the children or youth. Helping the children take down some of their walls of fear is a way to open their doors to receive God. This is a step that is sometimes left out by pastoral visitors.

There is a tendency among pastoral caregivers to arrive in the waiting room, greet the child, ask if he or she is afraid, hear the child say, "No," and then focus on the parents. This is sometimes improved upon when pastoral visitors make a comment intended to normalize or legitimize a child's fear. However, a more child-centered pastoral care might proceed on at least two levels. The first is the level of information. What does the child actually expect to happen? An open-ended question such as, "Can you tell me what you think is going to happen to you today?" will usually elicit ideas and expectations. The pastoral warning flags should arise when the child cannot give an answer at all, if the answer is obviously inappropriate, or if the parents answer before the child has an opportunity to speak. Pastoral caregivers who have had surgery or who have been through the experience as a waiting family member may find it helpful to do some self-disclosure. One might verbally walk the child through what can be expected after being called to the operating room. Information is one way in which children cope with new experiences, and the pastor may be able to provide this information. What happened to you? What did the room look like? What was the first thing that happened when you got to the operating room? What was the first thing you remember when you woke up? Pastoral caregivers who intend to do a great deal of hospital visiting or who have not had a personal experience of surgery may find it helpful (before there is a need) to make an appointment with the surgical charge nurse and ask for a guided tour so that they can then better prepare children for the experience.

Children who make a substantive answer to the question about their expectations or who have talked through this with the pastor may be ready to talk on an emotional level. Pastoral caregivers might invite them to move to that deeper level with some personal sharing of experience: "When I was waiting for surgery, I was feeling . . ." and an open-ended follow-up question such as, "I wonder what is going on inside you right now?" Normalizing the fears is a good thing to do; being anxious before surgery is a perfectly reasonable feeling. Dealing with their emotions is a perfectly reasonable thing for a pastoral caregiver to do. It is not all that we are about, however, and at some point a pastoral visit can move into talking about God. How and when that transition happens is sensed more intuitively in the moment than by any clear signals. I favor open-ended questions that portray God as immanent and responsive: "What would you like to hear from God this morning?" or "I am wondering if you have talked with God about your surgery?" are ways of phrasing this.

Some children have been taught not to show fear, and pastoral caregivers may even encounter parents who will make comments such as, "He is not afraid, are you?" How can a child answer truthfully in the face of such parental expectations? Unlike inpatient areas in a hospital, in a surgical waiting room it will be virtually impossible to ask parents to leave while you have a private conversation with the child. Situations where the child has been "set up" by a parent are difficult places in which to minister. One response might be to respond directly to the child, essentially ignoring the parental remark, and say that if he is afraid, that is okay, but that many times people, even adults, are afraid and that is okay too. Jesus was afraid before he went through a big experience (recalling the night of agony in the garden), and his disciples were afraid in the boat when the high wind and big waves came up. What Jesus did then was pray. The pastoral visitor might then slip right into a prayer with the child and family. In cases where the children have a prior relationship with the pastoral visitor, they will trust what is said to them and draw strength from it, even as they hold it in tension with what a parent has told them.

Many pastoral caregivers use prayer as a way to end a visit. It is the last thing we do before we leave a room. The advantage is that it can sum up all that has gone before and lift it up to God. The disadvantage is that it can be misinterpreted as a signal that "I am about to leave!" I want to suggest that prayer need not be offered out of a sense of duty or routine; it is rather our desire to communicate with God. It is possible that if the prayer is deferred until the end of the visit, the pastoral caregiver may find that the surgical team has arrived early, preempting the prayer! The prayer now competes with the careplan: the child is distracted, the surgical team is interested in keeping to their pace, and the parents have completely forgotten that the pastoral caregiver exists. What to do in this case? One option is to have the prayer sooner rather than later. For instance, say to the child after talking about his or her feelings, "How about if we say a prayer to God about all of this?"

The content of the prayer will largely be informed by the pastoral caregiver's own religious tradition. Certainly it is good to include any specific feelings the child has named and any requests for God that the child has indicated. I find it helpful to pick *one* biblical image, such as Jesus calming the storm and the disciples' fears, and weave that into what has come out of our conversation. I also include in my prayer some words asking for God's blessing and guidance for the child's surgeon and the surgical team. As a chaplain I have learned how much the surgical team appreciates being included in the prayers. More important, it helps the child view them as being included in the circle, along with family and God. If the pastoral caregiver prayed for the doctors and nurses too, then they must be okay.

GUILTY FEELINGS

Guilt is a common feeling that anyone who provides pastoral care to children and youth will encounter:

> Sheila had an automobile accident while driving her parents' car without their permission or knowledge while they were away from the house. She sustained relatively minor physical injuries and was alert and talking in the emergency department. Upon her parents' arrival, the chaplain told Sheila that her parents were coming in. She responded, "Oh, no! I cannot face them now."

Guilty feelings, such as those expressed by Sheila, are given voice in a variety of events involving children. They also occur in more chronic or long-term situations as well, although they then tend to be feelings voiced by the parents. In an acute event, it is also quite likely that one will encounter them being spoken by the child. For this reason, I choose to deal with them at this point. Such feelings are very powerful ones, but also somewhat complex. Understanding some of the dynamics of guilt is important in considering how one might frame a pastoral response to the child.

When life experiences do not match our expectations, one response is to assume that we are somehow at fault. Some persons will assume a large share of blame for a situation. This is a very common experience when a child's life has changes. A child will believe, and sometimes say, "It is my fault that . . ." The sentence may be completed by a wide variety of endings ranging from "my parents are divorcing" to "I wrecked the car" or "I did not watch my brother closely enough," all of which are a child's assumption of guilt for an event.

Most pastoral caregivers will be able to remember instances in which people expressed guilty feelings due to something that was genuinely their fault and also times when people expressed guilty feelings for insignificant events. Sometimes people have guilty feelings they cannot let go of, no matter how many times they have been assured that there is no problem. What we call "guilt" can be what is termed "appropriate guilt." These are feelings that arise because a person's actions have violated that person's ideas about what is right and have harmed that person or another in some way. Guilty feelings can also be what is sometimes called "inappropriate guilt." This includes feeling guilty for events that are not truly our responsibility or feeling guilty after having been forgiven or assured that we were not at fault. Or they may arise because feeling bad about ourselves actually provides some benefit to us. They also arise when an acute event causes an old memory of our own to resurface, usually a memory of a time when we were made to feel guilty. Those resurfaced feelings can be so strong that they dictate how we respond to the present, acute situation.

Being able to recognize these two forms of guilt is important for pastoral caregivers because the response to each is different. Well-adjusted, mature adults experience appropriate guilt precisely because they are psychologically mature: they have an internal "code of ethics" and when they violate it, they experience guilty feelings. Inappropriate guilt does not arise from a mature psyche—and for that very reason is commonly experienced by children and youth. A stereotypical example is a child feeling responsible for a parent's divorce or disease.

This is not to say that children do not experience appropriate guilt simply because they are too young. Children as young as two or three years of age have some understanding of right and wrong. Toddlers who push the boundaries of behavior are learning just how far they can go before the parents step in with the limit. Their internal code of ethics is in its earliest stages of formation, but they can experience guilt after being reprimanded for hitting someone they love, such as a parent. Inappropriate guilt, however, is a feeling pastoral caregivers may expect to encounter and which may be regarded as age appropriate.

Pastoral caregivers can help persons move through appropriate guilt by helping them openly name what event, word, or thought violated this internal code of ethics. What has been done wrong, who has been hurt, and how? Naming requires more than simply having someone say, "I did drugs the other night and it was wrong!" Naming is a process that the pastor can help the person move through by exploring how the behavior has hurt people. To use this example, one can ask these questions: How do drugs harm the body, which is a gift of God? How has this drug use affected the lives of others, such as parents or friends? If this person was doing drugs with another friend, how has he or she helped that person hurt others, given the strength in numbers of doing drugs together?

This is essential because the next step is to name the emotion. Guilt is assuaged only when one is sorry or contrite for one's action. Only when the full impact of the action has been thoroughly explored and named can the person feel the fullest sorrow for the action. Those feelings of sorrow find expression in confession. Here, different faith groups will have different practices and beliefs ranging from formal rites of reconciliation presided over by a clergyperson to the private words of confession one says silently to God. The children's pastoral caregiver can outline how this process is handled in their tradition.

What God is far more interested in celebrating is not the guilt, sorrow, or confession, but that this process leads to a changed life. The final step of this process is amendment of life. This includes making right, when possible, whatever has created the guilty feelings in the first place. It also includes some exploration of how life will be different in the future. The pastoral caregiver can help children and youth understand this best by asking questions. "If this were to happen to you again tomorrow, what would you do differently?" Responses of "I do not know" can be responded to with an invitation to name all the possible options (and maybe even "priming the pump" by naming a few for the youth) and then exploring which one they would like to use as their first line of defense in the future.

In doing pastoral care with children, one does not always encounter appropriate guilt (even among their parents). Adults often do or say something that does not violate an internal code they have worked to establish, but does violate something they learned when they were children. Some children learn that it is not safe to express deep feelings openly in front of their parents. For example, boys are frequently taught that it is inappropriate to cry openly. When something happens to them later on that makes them cry (to use that example), they will feel guilt for having done something wrong. The youth did not go against one of their values or principles; they went against something someone else gave them which they never chose to discard or own.

Children and youth have generally not developed an internal set of rules that they live by; their principles are adopted, largely without examination, from adults with whom they have frequent contact. Part of the work of adolescence is reflecting on those principles and choosing to discard them or own them. To the extent that this work is unfinished, the child or youth is likely to experience inappropriate guilt. Moving someone through the steps of naming the wrong thought or behavior, confessing it in some way, and making amends will not work. The fact that someone continues to hang on to guilty feelings after having been through that process is itself a strong sign that they are feeling inappropriate guilt. Younger children may need multiple reassurances that an event is not their fault, and the pastoral caregiver needs to understand that, for children, continually hanging on to guilty feelings is age appropriate and normal. As they grow older, they may be able to look back and put their understanding of an event in a different context as they realize they did not cause someone to get cancer or to die. By contrast, older youth who express such feelings may need to be invited by the pastor to deal with them, as they then serve as a marker for unresolved issues.

Adults who express inappropriate or childish guilt are probably in need of therapeutic counseling to move them through it. On the other hand, there is nothing inappropriate about children experiencing childish guilt. For their current state of development, this is perfectly acceptable. The question is, how to approach the child? A gentle confrontation that redirects the child's thinking may be in order. ("You know, your brother fell down the steps and broke his arm because he tripped, not because you yelled at him. You still seem pretty upset—tell me how you and your brother get along.") Here the child's view of reality is gently redirected, and then the pastoral caregiver moves the issue away from the initial guilt feeling ("My brother broke his arm and it is my fault because I yelled at him") toward what the pastoral caregiver believes is the genuine and underlying issue (the sibling relationship). The real problem may not be solved, as parents divorcing may not change their minds solely because it troubles their child, nor will sibling rivalry disappear. Having been heard by the pastoral caregiver, though, the child's guilty feelings may lessen, and the door may be opened to begin a longer-term relationship with the child or with the family as a whole.

> Kenneth, a pastor in his midfifties, tearfully related a childhood experience that revealed emotional neglect and physical abuse by his parents while he was a young boy. At the end of his story, his facial expression softened and he said, "And a long time ago, I forgave them."

Forgiveness is a process, and it can be rushed. This is true whether the process began with appropriate, mature guilt or childish guilt. It is possible to forgive too soon. Forgiveness that comes "too soon" is an intellectual decision. The roots of it lie in self-defense. Someone has hurt us severely; rather than experience feelings of hurt and anger toward this person, we cut off feeling the emotions connected to the hurt by forgiving the offender. Then we need not feel guilty about our angry feelings at someone we were or want to be emotionally close to. The problem, of course, is that this merely covers up a hurt within us. Think for a moment about a physical wound. Wounds that are covered for long periods of time with debris and dirt will fester and create a more serious problem than wounds that are open and can be cleaned easily. So it is also with emotional wounds. The important issue is to remember to never, ever rush children or youth to forgiveness. They need time to name the problem, look at its effects, feel sorrow, and look at future actions. Rarely can so much ground be covered in a single conversation.

ANGER

It goes without saying that no one enjoys being angry, and the church historically has not encouraged people to feel or express their anger. This is not a plea to encourage children to histrionic displays whenever the situation does not go their way. What is important is to provide a safe place for children to discover and express appropriate, righteous anger and not insist on forgiveness. You may even have to help them name the feeling, since it may well involve being angry at a parent, stepparent, or sibling—someone with whom it is not permissible to be angry. A door opener such as, "Gee, I would be really, really mad if someone did that to me!" may encourage them to name whatever emotion they are feeling.

After the child is able to name the feelings, then you can decide to move on to the religious dimension. This will be covered more fully in the chapter on mental health issues, but an opening question such as, "How do you suppose God feels about what has happened?" is a way to broach this subject. What kind of a response God may want from us can be a goal for future discussion. This is obviously a lengthy process, which cannot be completed in a single conversation.

Nonaccidental Trauma: Their Anger and Yours

Physical and sexual abuse of children remains all too common in society. Pastoral caregivers are in a prime position to notice when abuse of any kind may be happening and to take steps to help children be safe. This is because of the tremendous entrée that pastoral persons have into the lives of families. Once inside (both literally and figuratively), the pastoral caregiver should be alert for the major dynamic of anger.

In many cases there is a strong desire to protect ourselves from the truth that child abuse does occur and think, "not in my congregation," but the sad truth is that it can happen anywhere. In my role as a hospital chaplain, I have been asked several times to baptize young children who have been shaken so severely that their brains are damaged. Sometimes the damage is so severe that they will die within a few hours. On some of those occasions, one of the family members standing around the bedside is the one who inflicted this horrible damage. I do not always know which person it is. They have no horns or cloven hooves; they look like you and me.

If children have been injured so severely as to require hospitalization, you may still be able to visit. If custody has been taken by the local children's services bureau, you may need to go through that office to secure permission to visit the children. Once inside the room, your visit can be guided in the same way that other pastoral visits with children occur. Play is an important way children express feelings and make sense out of what has happened to them. Provide an emotionally safe place for this to occur. If there are marks or bandages visible on their bodies, do not be afraid to gently ask about them ("Can you tell me what happened to your arm, Sophie?"). Children know these are visible; if you do not comment on them, children may think they are unsightly or ugly. There should not be a two-headed purple monster that no one is talking about in the room! Failing to comment on the obvious suggests that it is too horrible to discuss. If they believe something about themselves is too horrible to be discussed openly, they will likely experience a sense of being dirty or unclean, unlovable, and cut off from God.

Anger is an emotion that you can simply expect to be present. The child may or may not be ready to talk about it, but you can provide places for it to come out ("I am wondering how you felt when that happened to you?"). Some children may feel bad (more accurately, guilty) about being angry at a parent, even if that parent has hurt them. They may need to be given permission to be angry and to express that anger.

This can be done very explicitly. You might share your own angry feelings toward a driver who ran a stop sign and caused a car accident. After doing so, an open-ended invitation can be made: "I am wondering if you feel something similar?" If they say that they are not feeling any anger, move on and do not dwell on what you think they should be feeling. It may be too soon, or they may not be good at talking about their feelings. Or they may not know you well enough at this point to open up. If you have the opportunity at a future date, you may wish to bring the question up again.

Some pastoral caregivers use Scripture to make their points, and certainly there are passages that cover anger. Rather than read a story about righteous anger out of the Bible to a child, tell the child the story from your memory as if it were a bedtime story. It will likely have a more significant impact than something read from a book. For that reason, a story from the Bible is a better choice than some of the psalms that deal with anger. They do not lend themselves to storytelling as well. If you choose to make use of Scripture with children, remember that they generally are concrete thinkers. After telling them the story, you will need to make it very clear why you told it. They may wonder why you told them about God's anger unless you clearly connect it to what they may be feeling.

The child is not the only person who may be feeling anger. Sometimes the pastoral caregiver must cope with his or her own anger. A month or so after my wife had a miscarriage, I was called to the emergency department to find that an infant who had been physically abused had been brought in. I sat down with the family and introduced myself, but I was quickly aware that I was so furious over what had happened that I could not function as a pastor to them, and I asked the social worker to take over for me. This event, with its parallel sense of injustice to our miscarriage, served as a trigger for my own feelings of grief, powerlessness, and indignation.

I cite this story as an example that it is important for pastoral caregivers to be aware of their own feelings. If these feelings are too much for you to effectively minister to a child or family, back away and provide some other pastoral support for the child or family. There are also times when it may not be possible to act as pastor to both the child and to all of the family members. Then it is time to ask an associate in the congregation or request that a pastoral caregiver from a nearby congregation take over for you. You may also need to find someone with whom you can process your feelings about such an event.

You may have the good fortune never to have this kind of experience touch you. That does not mean that it does not occur or that there is no way that you can still provide pastoral care for children who do experience such trauma. For example, when a child comes to the hospital within seventy-two hours of suspected or probable sexual abuse, the underwear will be taken. If the visit is within twenty-four hours, all of the clothing will be taken and sent away for laboratory analysis as forensic evidence. This means the hospital probably has no clothing to give the child to wear home other than the traditional hospital gown, which is short and does not fully close in the back, and, perhaps, a pair of pajama bottoms.

Congregations and pastoral caregivers might adopt a hospital and provide a supply of new underwear, sweatpants, and T-shirts (that are not white nor see-through). With these clothes, children may leave with some dignity, without making it clear that they have just come from a hospital, which could invite intrusive questions. An outreach project such as this can be an excellent way to provide comfort and care to children and to teach them that there are people who simply care about them without even meeting them. You might begin such a project by inquiring in the social work or emergency departments in a local hospital how they respond to this need and if they could use your efforts.

VISITING IN ACUTE CARE AREAS

As a pastoral caregiver, your presence in the emergency department or an intensive care unit will usually be welcomed by the staff. The staff will generally see your role as taking care of the family. While this is often in large measure a reasonable vision of your role, pastors ought not to let someone else define their role for them. The staff will likely view you as another professional and, therefore, as someone less likely to become a histrionic adult patient that would then need their care. This may mean that you will have access to be with the child when no one else, including the parents, is able to do so. Virtually no one, however, including pastoral persons, should be allowed to remain present with a child during a resuscitation effort.

Whether or not parents should be present during resuscitations is a matter of some debate, although the consensus is generally against it at present. So long as this is the case, nurses or other hospital personnel may ask you to help them by taking family members to a nearby room, out of sight and hearing from the trauma rooms. Family members may be more or less willing to do that, and there have been some occasions when having a family member present is soothing for the child and less stressful for the parent. If you find yourself in this situation, use your judgment after watching the scene. Is the parent actively seeking to soothe or respond to the child? Does the parent manage to keep out of the way? Will watching these procedures itself be a source of trauma for the family later on? How are the staff reacting to family presence? If the family member is providing a sense of comfort to the child and is able to "handle" being in the room, it may be that the parent should remain. As the child's pastor, you may need to be advocate and voice if staff ask the family member to leave and you believe this is not in the child's best interest. Remember that pastoral care is also about being the voice of the voiceless ones. That needs to be balanced with respect for other professionals, and although it may seem helpful for the family to remain, the staff may need to do or say something for which it would be best if the family were not present. Advocate for the child as you feel you need to, but remember it is the hospital staff who ultimately control what happens.

There are likely to be some periods of waiting, such as while waiting for X rays to be developed, or waiting to go to radiology, or waiting for the patient to be assigned a room, during which you could visit with the child. Seek out the child's nurse; in a trauma case, seek a nurse who is at or near the door of the trauma room and who is not obviously busy. Let the nurse know your relationship in terms of the patient ("I am Gina's priest"), rather than the family ("I am here with the Hernandez family"), and ask if you can speak to her briefly. If there are rituals that your religious tradition uses at such times, such as anointing, state succinctly that it is an important part of religious care in the patient's tradition. Having thus gained access to the patient, know that hearing is the sense that functions even when others are diminished. Always assume the patient can hear you, and speak or pray directly into the ear. If the patient is conscious, ask if there is anything you should tell the parents (or whomever you are with). Let the patient know who is in the waiting room. If the family has not yet spent time with the child, a word to a nurse as you leave—"How soon do you expect the parents to be able to come in?"—will either get you a concrete answer in minutes or serve as a reminder to the staff that the parents have not yet been in and that they are waiting and anxious to visit their child.

Chapter 4

Pastoral Issues in Chronic Care

Although, compared to adults, children tend to become sicker faster, and to recover more quickly, children must also cope with a variety of conditions that are long term. Such conditions may take many forms, from asthma and diabetes, which are relatively mild and can be well controlled by the child and family, to more serious conditions such as cystic fibrosis, leukemia, and a wide range of developmental impairments. These conditions are usually called "chronic," which will be used here to refer to any disease or condition with which a child must cope for more than several months. The adults in the family constellation cannot help but be affected by what has occurred in the child. Their spiritual care, however, will largely be similar to pastoral care of other adults, and hence most pastoral caregivers feel on somewhat familiar ground. Pastoral caregivers have a wealth of spiritual care to contribute to the child or youth, and this is the focus of this chapter.

Although being told you have been diagnosed with a long-term condition is an event, living with it is a process with many stops along the way. Having a sense of what is to come allows the pastoral caregiver to outline the future for the child, which may help normalize some of the anxiety. It also allows caregivers to ask questions that have to do with what the child is experiencing.

No child or family moves through the course of any condition as if following the same road map as all other children with the same condition. There is no evolutionary sequence to describe what they will be experiencing at a given time. At the same time, there are several stops along the journey that many patients and families make, and it is worth noting some of them.

Diagnosis means giving a name to something; it is a title in search of subject matter to stand beneath it. Many diagnoses have such power that the family or teen may not hear anything that follows ("Your son has Burkitt's lymphoma"). At some point, many people seek information and attempt to learn all they can about the disease, its treatment, and course. This is to be affirmed; better-informed patients and families make better decisions. This only becomes a block when people become stuck there and have difficulties in making decisions or in maintaining relationships (both interpersonal relationships or between themselves and God).

At some point a new rhythm of life emerges. It may happen quickly once children learn to control their sugar intake and take their insulin. Or it may take a longer time, adjusting to many outpatient treatments and their side effects. This new rhythm of life provides an opportunity to ask the child or teen to reflect: how is life different from before?

Children and teenagers I have known whose conditions have been terminal, frequently conceive of their futures differently than do adults. Adults tend to see such conditions as leading to an early death. When one's own child is involved, it is difficult to push that thought out of one's mind. Children, whose own concept of death at that age means that they do not regard it as a permanent condition, often lack the fear that adults experience. Teenagers may share the adult view around the time of diagnosis but tend to be caught up in more immediate concerns. Like their more healthy counterparts, they deal with short-term concerns. In this case, it means frequently focusing on such things as the immediate treatment rather than taking a longer-term view. In this case, focusing on the immediate protects them from many of the feelings that their parents experience.

The pastoral implication here is as it has always been: be with the person where they are. In the case of a teenager with a chronic condition, that means focusing on the teen's concerns and not projecting the pastoral caregiver's own fears and emotions onto the youth:

> Lela was an eighteen-year-old with a solid tumor. When her local pastor entered her room and asked how she was doing, Lela rolled her eyes and said, "I have been puking all day long. It is nasty. It is bright and it is green and it has chunks in it."

The pastor began to turn a shade of green herself at this point. Nevertheless, she responded, "Sounds like a pretty crummy day. It is pretty nasty when the drugs that are supposed to help you make you puke interesting colors!"

This vignette illustrates several things. First, chronic conditions are often viewed by children and youth as nuisances rather than as something that will kill them. Certainly there are times when they are afraid, but do not assume this to be their overriding theme. Second, children and teenagers are often more matter-of-fact about what they experience than we might expect. The pastor in this vignette managed to set aside her own assumptions and fears about the disease. She is tracking the patient's concern and staying focused on the teenager. The ability to do this, to *listen* to a nine-year-old rehearse what it is like to inject himself with insulin or an eighteen-year-old talk about the unpleasant side effects of chemotherapy, is essential to providing pastoral care to children and teenagers.

Pastoral care also means helping people be aware of who they *are*. Having a disease or condition with a *name* changes one's identity. One sees himself or herself as the disease ("I am a diabetic"). To be this reductionistic is not good or bad, but it reflects how a condition fiddles with one's identity as a person. To a greater or lesser extent, it changes one's sense of self. The fundamental pastoral question, of course, is the extent to which it alters one's sense of being God's child.

Pastoral relationships are relationships of trust, built upon speaking the truth to one another as it is known. Honesty with children about their condition is to be most strongly encouraged. Information needs to be delivered at a level that they can understand. Recall that the very first step in human development (according to Erikson) is to negotiate the basic issue of trust versus mistrust. To fail to deal honestly with children or teens about their condition will cause developmental regression. A breach of this trust, however perceived, will slow down every pastoral process. The capacity to cope is directly linked with honesty in the pastoral relationship. Failing to be honest with children takes more work in the long run; old developmental ground must be recovered. Most adults, parents, and pastoral caregivers alike want to protect children. The healthiest way to do this is to speak genuinely and truthfully.

The way in which our culture views persons who have chronic medical needs has changed over the years. The pastoral implication, not surprisingly, is that how pastoral caregivers view illness and their role has changed as well. In my early pastoral training, this topic was covered under the title of perpetual grief. That was the dominant paradigm for describing the patient's and family's response to chronic conditions. To live with a chronic condition was somehow to be less than fully alive, a situation of loss that was to be grieved and mourned. A more contemporary paradigm is, "any anatomical or physiological impairment that interferes with the individual's ability to function fully in the environment" (Fulton and Moore, 1995, p. 224). The pastoral caregiver's role formerly was to help the family, and perhaps the child, cope with the loss of their expectations, and usually, to prepare for the child's death. Presently, the pastoral role has shifted to focus upon the child's relationship with God and with other people. This is spiritual friendship. Being the spiritual friend of children or youth means being someone who meets them *on their terms*, to be their companion, and to do this for the purpose of helping them grow in their experiences of God.

SPIRITUAL FRIENDSHIP

Chronic conditions last for a long time, and sometimes the child or youth appears to be feeling quite well. There is a tendency to assume that pastoral needs are fewer or nonexistent. A common response is to drastically reduce, or even terminate, the number of pastoral contacts that are made with the child:

> In the midst of playing a card game with Henedine, she looked at me and said, "You are here all the time. How come Pastor John does not come any more?" I was surprised because I knew that this child's pastor had been coming almost daily since the bike accident put her in the intensive care unit. She had been on the regular floor for several days. Her mother nodded in confirmation explaining, "I think maybe he believes we are going to leave here in two weeks and everything will be

normal again. He forgets that we have to go to rehab and learn how to walk before she can go back to school." A few hours later, I checked the clergy sign-in books and the family's perception was correct. While Henedine was in ICU the pastor visited at least daily. He had only visited once since she was moved to a regular room.

As Henedine's mother implies, the girl's condition has improved a great deal. There is still a very long way to go, however, and her sense of being "forgotten" suggests that there are still some issues that she believes might be resolved with pastoral care. Similar complaints have been voiced by parents whose child is in a newborn intensive care unit for eight to ten weeks, by youth recovering from bicycle accidents, and by children with spina bifida. When there is a crisis, their pastoral caregivers are right there with them. When the acute condition fades, or at least when the emotional intensity begins to lessen and life appears to return to normal, pastoral care frequently fades into the background. The decreasing attention from pastoral caregivers is not malicious, and often unintentional. Frequently, it is due to the complex array of tasks that face ordained pastoral caregivers, as well as the needs of other individuals in a congregation that have suddenly become acute. As the child's ongoing condition returns to its more typical state, pastoral caregivers may be tempted to believe that this means there are no longer needs to be addressed. How does one provide for ongoing pastoral needs outside of a hospital? What do children and youth need when everything appears to be normal, or at least better than it was?

Typically, if the nature of the child's condition is maintenance, then the character of the pastoral visit can be maintenance as well. Resist self-imposed pressures for every visit to reach a deep level of intimacy. Pastoral care, especially with children, that effectively communicates God's love and God's abiding presence will seek its own level more often than not.

Maintenance pastoral care has as its goal maintaining relationships between children and God, the congregation, and the pastoral caregiver. This builds the foundation so that when there is an acute event or significant decisions need to be made, the pastoral person already has a trust-filled and ongoing relationship with the child an ' family. Such visits have an element of "checking in" about them. This also serves to overcome the feelings of isolation from a worshiping community that may come as a result of the child's condition.

The pastoral caregiver might suggest to a school-age child that they visit and perhaps play a game for a little while. With an adolescent, it may take the form of an invitation to go out for a pizza and talk about football or band or hobbies. Simple, casual inquiries into "how it is going" with the condition are all that is required. It might be worth inquiring if the condition has been keeping the child from doing something. Youth will generally signal when they have questions or are ready to talk about a particular issue in depth. Younger children will reveal some of this through play. Such conversations can proceed as with any other pastoral talk.

The Ministry of Introduction

One of this book's themes, which should be evident by now, is the *isolating nature of illness.* Unique contributions by pastoral caregivers bring an end to isolation. A ministry of presence creates community. There is another kind of community that caregivers can facilitate, and that is relationships between children and youth who share similar conditions. Know your congregation so that when a child is diagnosed with a condition, you may be able to link the child up with another child experiencing the same condition.

It is common for someone with a condition in its early stages to think that he or she is the only person having this experience. A good pastoral question is, "Do you know anyone else who has this condition?" This question accomplishes two things. First, it reveals a potential support community or alerts the pastoral caregiver to gaps in the continuum of care. Second, the question is a reality check. The person may know someone else with the same disease, but may not have an accurate perception of what their own course may be like. If the person seems to have extreme views demonstrated by exaggerating or minimizing the condition or the treatment, then it is a signal to educate. Pastoral caregivers might help prepare a list of questions to ask a physician or others who have the same condition.

Knowing the children and youth in your congregation well enough to make introductions is a wonderful level of knowledge to have reached. With this knowledge comes a measure of responsibility. Some persons who have their condition under control do not want to meet with newly diagnosed persons. It brings back difficult memories of when and how they experienced a life change. Or they simply do not have the energy nor the relational skills to invest. Choose your referrals wisely. Neither person should show signs of becoming emotionally dependent upon the other. When a child seems interested in meeting or talking with others who are in the same position, this is your permission to share names and perhaps telephone numbers. Always approach the child who has had the condition for some time first, and ask if he or she would be willing to contact someone you know who has just been diagnosed. Then you can share the child's name and any other information.

The hospital, clinic, or physician's practice to which the child or youth belongs may already have such a group in place. The underground network of persons who have a chronic condition is often surprisingly extensive. The sudden change in condition of a member of such a group or the death of a member frequently produces a ripple effect throughout the community of kids who share that condition. Ask them how others they know are doing. Pay attention to the changes in the conditions of those known to you. A death of another child triggers questions and fears in many others.

Contemplative Prayer

There is more to spiritual friendship than simply playing and being friendly with children or youth. "Wasting time" with God is a way of finding peace in life. Although they will no doubt feel cared for at some level, this is a friendship with a difference. And that difference is the attention the pastoral caregiver pays to helping them forge and maintain a relationship with God. Children and teenagers still operate on a level that allows some mystery and some fantasy. Pastoral caregivers can make use of this state of their development by suggesting some different, perhaps untraditional, ways of relating to God. Children are quite willing to accept and experiment with new ways of praying, which fall under the category of wasting time with God. This has been especially true after someone has reached the point of frustration: "I have been praying to God, but it is like God does not hear—I am still diabetic!" When youth can give voice to that frustration, it is a signal that they are open to trying something a little different. They are ready to simply be with God. For those few minutes, they can be whole and healthy just because they are with God. Having suggested this to a youth, the pastoral caregiver can almost hear the youngster's next statement: "But what happens when I am done praying? I am not cured, am I?" To which I would respond honestly, "No, you will not be cured. But others your age who have spent time with God like this often come away feeling more relaxed or more at peace."

Rethinking Prayer and Healing

Prayer or meditation puts us in the presence of God and contributes to our wholeness and, therefore, also to our health. This was one of the first lessons that chaplaincy taught me, and it has become the premise from which much of my prayer life and preaching now grows. Human life is imperfect and always has some brokenness. I think we have something to gain from living out a relationship with God, who alone is whole and perfect. Our word health comes from an Old English word *hal*, which means whole; put another way, that which makes us whole makes us healthy again.

People who have a religious or spiritual bent often know this intuitively, but this seems to be borne out in recent medical literature. There is a growing body of articles in the medical and pastoral care literature that reflects the current interest in exploring the relationship between health and prayer. Introducing a child to some form of prayer, in addition to any medical intervention, is likely to be more effective in producing a whole child than simply educating him or her about the disease process.

Information is an important coping mechanism and can lead to decisions for healthy behaviors. While learning about a disease is important, it is not in itself healing. There are other levels of coping and functioning that are deeper than that of information. What the pastoral caregiver wants to be able to do is to help the children or youth tap into their well of mystery and their ability to step outside the bounds of what is rational. Children and youth can be encouraged to use their imaginations, not to remove the disease, which may not be possible, but to approach wholeness.

Understanding prayer in this way calls for thinking about prayer differently than many adults are accustomed to doing. In the United States near the end of the twentieth century, we have been trained by the Enlightenment to approach our world in a rational, scientific, and technological way. It can be difficult to set that approach aside and look at other ideas. The world of the writers of Scripture was one in which God did amazing things. It was a pre-scientific world, with none of the language of science. The Bible is not a serious science textbook but one that explores how God loves people and how we can respond to God. The writers of Scripture remind us that our own visions, dreams, and individual prayers play a vital role in our response to God. Being able to help children and youth tap into their abilities to experience God in those ways promotes their healing.

Making this shift in thinking has to begin inside the pastoral caregiver before it can be offered to the children and youth in our care. The following outlines a new way of thinking about prayer that can enrich how you help children and youth approach God. What follows is important because it serves as the background for the approaches to working with children and youth that are presented.

In our rational approach to reality, there are poles of thought that can roughly be called traditionally Western and Eastern. I do not believe that either is completely correct, but I do believe that the two can inform each other. In the Eastern view of life, everything is somehow connected and is circular. Eastern thought is very comfortable with paradox. In a religious example, this is being able to hold in tension one's faith in a good God and behold the reality of disease and abuse, accepting the mystery of being unable to understand fully. In Eastern thought, persons are seen as total beings, rather than the more Western view of the body as a machine. In the Eastern view, everything has a place and is somehow connected. This includes disease. Illness is, as I have said, a self-*ish* experience. It is, after all, what happens to, or wells up within, my body, and I carry these implications throughout my life. Therefore, I have some responsibility for how I respond to illness and how I live with it. What I do affects my disease process. Most obviously, I choose to take my medicine, to see my physician, or *not*. The Eastern philosophy regards love as essential. A growing body of evidence coming out of coronary care units has examined the rate of marital problems among those who have cardiac events, and the findings suggest that people really do die of broken hearts. The inability to love, either because one has no mate or because there is not a healthy relationship with a mate, may contribute to some cardiac problems.

We in the West, however, have been trained to think in a very logical, step-by-step fashion. This is not necessarily wrong, but it does lead to problems when it is the only type of thinking that gets done! In this view, a paradox is seen as something that needs to be resolved and explained. The so-called Age of Enlightenment, during the fourteenth through eighteenth centuries in Europe, sought to categorize and label every aspect of the world. This approach, although not inherently bad, does have a demonic side. By demonic, I mean that when someone is reduced to an action, or reduced to a disease, then part of one's humanity has been denied. Disease is seen as coming from outside the body. When that is the picture of disease, then individuals are absolved from responsibility for how they live with it. Disease is "unnatural" and, therefore, is an invasion into our bodies, our lifestyles, our childhoods. It is something against which we should struggle. Last, Western science has largely ignored love as a power that can effect change.

None of the techniques that follow are in the least original; the reader will recognize an interest in dreams and visions that goes back to the Hebrew Scriptures and is carried through such Christian giants as St. John of the Cross, Theresa of Avila, and Julian of Norwich. Today, such talk of dreams is frequently dismissed as unscientific. These writers, also known as mystics, are often regarded as so much navel-gazing by the majority of persons in a congregation and, hence, are largely unknown except by a few. The energy and richness of symbols that an Eastern spirituality has to offer makes for some ideal offerings. I advocate suggesting these to older school-age children and youth, especially those with chronic illness or long-term recoveries from trauma.

Practicing Contemplative Prayer During Pastoral Visits

The simplest of these prayer techniques is the relaxation response. Suggest that the youth pick a word or phrase that has meaning. A simple one to suggest is, "Lord, be with me" or simply the name "Jesus." Suggest that they close their eyes to eliminate distractions and begin to breathe in and out slowly. Repeat the word or phrase with each inhalation. Distractions will certainly come—rather than fight them or try to ignore them, suggest that the youth acknowledge them ("Oh, that is my dog barking") and then move on. Suggest that this be done for a limited amount of time each day. In the beginning, one or two minutes every few hours is reasonable.

Some people are simply strongly vision oriented and may find it very difficult to relax with only a word or phrase going through their minds. Focusing attention on an object such as a flower or candle or religious picture may help.

Guided imagery or imaginary journeys are another step up in sophistication. Quite a few of the teenagers who I have talked to on the adolescent psychiatric unit have been very open to such imaginary journeys. The conversations we have had as follow-ups to their journeys have been some of the most depth-filled and vulnerable conversations I have ever had. Offer to take the youth on an imaginary journey when you find that the youth has difficulty engaging an issue directly. It may be easier to talk about it in the safe place to which the journey takes the youth or after returning from the safe place. Another time such a suggestion can be made part of a pastoral visit is when the pastoral caregiver finds the youth experiencing pain, whether or not that pain is relieved by drugs. Taking someone on an imaginary journey is not difficult and requires only two things. The first is trust, and the second is undisturbed time.

A trust-filled relationship must be established between the youth and the pastoral caregiver. In agreeing to be led by you on an imaginary journey, the child or youth is opening up one side of the brain to you, and it is vital that the pastoral caregiver not manipulate the child into feeling or experiencing something that is not authentically there. This trustful openness serves to inspire a sense of awe and humility in approaching the task of leading such a journey. I do not write this to discourage you from offering this way of being with God when you feel it is appropriate. It is very important that you begin a journey having a solid appreciation for the level of responsibility you have taken.

The second requirement is a place and time with the youth when you are both undisturbed. Music playing quietly in the background is helpful. This promotes a relaxed atmosphere. It will also mask noises which might otherwise distract you or the child, and it creates some further privacy for any follow-up conversation you might have by preventing others from hearing the two of you clearly.

When these two conditions have been met, you are ready to begin the journey. I usually ask, "Do you have a place that is really special to you? Someplace where you like to go and feel really comfortable? You do not have to tell me where it is; I just want to know if you have one." If they do not have such a place, I invite them to create one with me as we begin and to imagine what it has in it. Are there trees? Birds? Animals? Is it a beach? Or a house on a quiet street? A family dinner full of laughter? Once they have a place, I invite the youth to close their eyes, and ask them to see their comfortable place. Ask them to go there in their minds with their eyes closed. Some time should be spent just being in that place and breathing slowly and evenly. The guide can then add some characters into the view; this could be family members or others important to an issue, or the pastor might ask the youth to visualize a particular character out of the Scriptures or even to visualize God or Jesus. The youth might be invited to talk to that character. After some time, the guide should say that it is time for the journey to end and that the youth should come back to the present time and place and when ready, open their eyes. An open-ended question to make sure the youth are all right is in order, and then ask how they felt about the people on the journey. How did the people respond to them? Were they judgmental, welcoming, or loving? Did they feel relaxed, safe, or scared?

The time to suggest this technique to youth who have a chronic condition is while they are feeling relatively well. This technique allows the youth to be near God's presence and perhaps to build or strengthen that relationship. Youth have found this kind of prayer helpful in dealing with the stress of a chronic condition and have used it as a way to talk to God about what is going on with them. After guiding the youth once or twice, the pastoral caregiver can remind the youth about using this technique alone. When the youth need some quiet time or when they want God to know what is going on, this is another way to express that to God directly.

Sometimes pain or anxiety attacks are sufficiently strong that a dialogue with youth is not possible. This does not necessarily mean that a pastoral visit is inappropriate. It is always worth beginning by inquiring whether the pain is controlled by medication. This question may be asked of teenagers directly; with younger children, one should ask the parents. One might ask the children or youth if they would like the pastoral caregiver to teach them a way to cope with, or to control, their pain or anxiety. Such a coping mechanism is meant to supplement, and never to replace, medically prescribed pain control. This technique begins again in a comfortable place, which the pastoral caregiver asks the youth to visualize. They are then led to a door that opens, and then they walk down four or five steps into an empty room. At this point, various options are possible depending upon the ages of the children and their level of articulation.

Tell them to see their pain in that room. Ask them to describe the pain. ("It looks like a big black monster with fangs and yellow teeth and it is looking right at me!") Sometimes I will ask what color their pain is. Most children who are experiencing pain at that time will choose red, orange, or yellow. I will ask them to see that color in their mind's eye. I then tell them to imagine that waves of ice blue water will wash over their red pain. This continues until the red is completely covered, after which they can remain in the room awhile longer before turning and walking back up the steps, through the door, and back to their guide.

Another related option, once they have been led into the empty room, is to say that the only item in the room is a machine with a big dial on the front. This dial controls pain levels. The guide can begin by asking where, between 1 and 10, the dial is set. Once the children give a number to their pain, then ask them to see themselves reaching out and turning that dial down one or two notches. Most children are not able to turn it down to zero and maintain that level. Many can turn it down part way and, after climbing the steps out of the room and returning to the present, report that their pain is less. As with the other techniques for guided imagery, this is something that the pastoral caregiver can teach the youth as one more tool available to deal with the condition.

Journaling is another form of prayer that may be suggested. This has the advantage of being available to a wider range of ages than guided imagery. Children and youth are inveterate diary-keepers; journaling is really just the adult name for this activity. With school-age children who may be unfamiliar with this or who find writing in a book too abstract, the pastoral caregiver may suggest that they write a letter to God each time rather than "Dear Journal, . . ."

The topics are limitless. Suggestions include the following. Do not let this list limit your thinking; be creative!

- What would you like to tell God today?
- Write a letter to yourself, saying what God might tell *you* in a letter.
- What would you like to hear from God right now?
- Suppose someone a few years younger (or older) had the same condition that you have; what would you tell that person about it?

At a clergy-spouse conference I attended some years ago, a physician who is married to a clergyperson told me, "I have never had anyone come to see me because he or she worked too hard. People come to me because they do not play hard enough!" The importance of play in our lives is not to be underestimated. Play is part of what being a child or youth is all about; children express who they really are most clearly when they are at play. There is value in the not-very-traditional ways of relating to God in this life, and there are times when words simply are not there or when words are not enough. There is a need to be able to approach God playfully, and the methods outlined in this chapter represent ways to do just that. Although we live in a technological and rational society, this does not mean that the pastoral caregiver must be bound by those cultural values. As pastoral persons, we are reminders of the limitless mystery and Being who is beyond all understanding.

DYNAMICS OF DEPRESSION AND GRIEF

Shortly after a diagnosis with lifelong and/or life-shortening implications, it is natural for children and youth to respond emotionally with depression. It may be mild or severe and be of short or long duration. This is quite natural, and the pastoral caregiver may take this as part of the process by which the child grieves the old ideas of life. In this sense, the old paradigm of grief was correct. To some extent they have experienced the death of a lifestyle. For this to be the sole guiding principle for pastoral care is to give it too much weight. The lives of children living with chronic conditions today are full and rich. However, it is worth knowing the basics of the dynamics of depression and grief so that when the pastoral caregiver does encounter them, they can be named for what they are.

There are dynamics of grief that may appear after a diagnosis is made which are related to mourning and which the pastoral caregiver may find useful in understanding what is taking place. Many persons today are familiar with Elisabeth Kübler-Ross's (1969) stages of grief. One should not take these as an evolutionary sequence, in which one must work through each stage, complete its tasks, and only then move on to the next. One of them may dominate a person's way of thinking at any given time, while the others are "in remission." The passage of time or, perhaps, a signal event may lead a child from one way of thinking into another. A boy whose condition does not permit extensive physical exertion may be mostly at peace with it until his playmates begin playing in baseball leagues. He might be angry that he cannot join with them, or he might bargain with God to be made like other kids in return for the child doing something for God's benefit later. The more children are likely to engage in magical thinking due to their development (generally, younger school-age children), the more bargaining is a likely scenario.

Some pastoral persons find such bargaining wrong. However, this type of response may be affirmed by pastoral caregivers for two reasons. First, it is developmentally appropriate for some ages, and to expect otherwise is to force children to be either more regressed or more advanced than they are. Second, Abraham himself bargained with God so that God would spare a city from the intended destruction (Genesis 18:23-33). Instead of condemning such ideas, pastoral caregivers can simply let them be or perhaps encourage the children to spin the thoughts out even further. What would you like from God? What would you be able to do that you cannot do today?

Each of the dominant ways of thinking that Kübler-Ross outlined may be explored with open-ended questions that allow the children to describe who God is for them, or what they would like from God, or what they would like to say to God. As noted earlier, depression shortly after diagnosis is common. So is hope for a miracle. This hope may or may not be expressed verbally by the child, and may bring with it a spiritual dilemma for the pastoral caregiver:

> Ira was an older teenager with a chronic respiratory disease. He developed an infection and was taken to the hospital. The physicians were quite frank with Ira and his family and stated they were not certain he would survive this infection but that if he did, it was only a matter of time before another opportunistic infection would arise, which with his damaged lungs, would kill him. The physicians asked Ira to think about what choices he wanted to make about his future care. In a conversation that evening with his pastoral caregiver, he asked the pastoral caregiver to pray for a miracle that not only would he survive this infection but that his lung condition be cured.

What is the appropriate pastoral response to the dilemma of being asked to share in the hope for a miraculous cure? Sometimes the best medical and scientific information is relatively clear and conflicts with a prayer intention. How does one balance that against a child's plea from the heart? How does a pastoral caregiver stand as a person of the truth and yet not hold out false hope?

One pastoral response is to gently acknowledge the hope that the pastoral caregiver hears. In this vignette, Ira expressed his hope openly. In some cases, it will be less explicit, but the pastoral caregiver may hear its expression by listening with the third ear. Some reflective comments such as, "Sounds as if you are asking God for a miracle. I am wondering if you are feeling desperate" or "I am wondering if you are feeling that a miracle is the only thing that will help you now," may open up a discussion about how the child sees the current reality and God's role in it.

A second response, which immediately follows the first, is to go ahead and make the prayer as requested. I believe that God wants to hear the prayers that are in our hearts. If it is a hope for a miracle, then so be it. I assume that God can see and hear beyond the literal words of the prayer and be touched by the anguish and desire for life that lie behind those words. I do not believe doing so holds out a false hope. There is a difference that I see between saying, "God will cure you if you ask," and "That is really what you want God to hear. Then let us tell God just that." In the first example, the pastoral caregiver speaks the mind of God and in the second, the pastoral person stands as an intermediary between the child and God. I see that difference as crucial. Offering the prayer that Ira wants uses prayer to tell God what is in his heart, rather than using the prayer time to teach Ira about God's will, God's timing, or anything else.

After praying as requested, then ask follow-up questions about how a youth such as Ira believes that God acts. How involved in the details of life does someone believe God is? What would the miracle look like? What will happen if God does not grant the request?

MAKING DECISIONS

Part of pastoral care is helping children and youth find their voices—to talk to God and to others about what is happening within them. This is one way the baptismal vow to respect the dignity of every human being is lived out. When there is a chronic condition, decisions may need to be made about future care. There comes a point when the youth needs to have a voice in those discussions. One of the tasks of adolescence is separating one's self from parents. When it occurs in the context of a child with long-term medical needs, this creates a pastoral issue. Just as parents may want to close in and protect the child and move forward with treatment, he or she may be in the midst of asserting himself or herself and want to make his or her own decisions.

A pastoral caregiver is in a position to help the youth articulate his or her needs and desires and be a participant in discussions regarding care. Sometimes the best way to care for the youth is to be an advocate with the parents or with members of the medical team. How far to go with this is a matter of balance depending on the age of the child. A seventeen- or eighteen-year-old deserves to have wishes about treatment heard and respected that a nine-year-old may not.

CARING FOR CHILDREN
WITH SEVERE CHRONIC CONDITIONS

Anna is a four-year-old with a seizure disorder who needs to take her own oxygen tank with her when she leaves the safety of her house. The bright lights in the church frequently trigger seizures, and she is also prone to infections. Attending church is a major ordeal for her parents and presents risks to Anna that they prefer not to take. Nonetheless, they would like Anna to be a baptized member of the church and to be as much a part of it as she can be.

Tyree is a sixteen-year-old with a genetic disease that is terminal. He has a very flat affect and does not sleep well at home. This leaves him with little energy. He does believe in God and attends a congregation when he feels up to it, perhaps once or twice a year. His church experience now comes primarily from watching televised shows at home.

These two cases illustrate the isolation that a child's chronic medical condition can bring about. Several challenges confront pastoral caregivers: how to facilitate these children doing all that they functionally can while making some allowances for what is beyond them, and how to bring the church to them when they cannot get out. In the context of spiritual friendship, the church emerges, as John Chrysostom's prayer says, "when two or three are gathered together . . ." God will be present there. The trust that will develop over time will help pastoral caregivers understand what the children's limits are. If the children are not living into the fullness that they might, the pastoral caregiver may gently suggest or challenge them to reach for another level.

I am frequently asked how difficult it is for children to cope with their own death. In general, I find they cope amazingly well. This is not to say that dying is easy when it involves children or that their last months or days are peaceful and gentle. The same resiliency, though, that helps many children recover from acute injuries can rise to help other children cope with their terminal condition. There are some special pastoral interventions that may help them face this event.

Dying children are still children and they need to play with their friends. This means not only their regular playmates or the youth they hang out with, but also their spiritual friends. If you have been in the habit of doing guided imagery, this is certainly worth continuing in two ways. The first is to use the pain machine image as a means of pain control. The second is to take them to their comfortable place, and then insert a path in it. They follow this path and it takes them to a new place. There they meet a family member who has already died (obviously, you need to ascertain who that might be beforehand—usually a grandparent or a pet). Afterward, ask them to describe, or, if they have the energy, to draw a picture and describe what this place was like. Focus in on what they were doing in this place. Children who have some idea of who they will be in heaven generally cope better with dying. Identity is a source of strength and comfort.

Chapter 5

Pastoral Care
and Mental Health Issues

Nowhere has health care reform changed in America as it has with mental health. When I first came to a new hospital position, the average length of stay on the adolescent psychiatric unit was twenty-one days. The focus was on treatment and most of the patient's time was spent in group therapy, individual therapy, and family sessions. Five years later, such units function in a very different way. The focus is primarily on crisis stabilization. To be admitted at present, one must be a danger to one's self or to others. In general, this means some sort of self-harm such as cutting on one's body, attempted suicide, or making serious statements about doing so and having the means at hand to make good on the threats. It may also mean having intentions of harming others. The average length of stay is about five days. On occasion, persons with serious eating disorders are admitted, though usually for a longer period. Although the day is still filled with group and individual therapy, the goal is not to treat the condition so much as to stabilize the child emotionally (and medically if necessary), to determine medications needed, and to locate local community-based treatment options. Treatment has shifted outside the hospital.

In a previous chapter, I advocated that pastoral visitors decide in advance who they intend to focus upon during a visit, either the child or the parents. When facing the prospect of doing pastoral work with teenagers who have a mental illness, I am going to refine that a bit more. In a conversation I had with a child psychiatrist about clergy visiting teenagers who had depression, the observation was made that *if clergy are uncomfortable with teenagers in general, then they should not visit them.* The psychiatrist's point is strongly made, and I hope it gives pastoral visitors some pause. Am I comfortable with teenagers in general? What do I hope to accomplish with my visit: do I want them to feel the church cares for them, or do I want to work with them and contribute to their healing process? If your answer is the latter, then by all means go ahead. If your answer leans more toward the former, you may be able to better spend your time visiting the parents and asking them to remember you to the teenager.

Throughout the rest of this book, I have tried to use an inclusive term, pastoral caregiver, to denote the person providing pastoral care, unless there was a sufficient reason to mandate that the visitor be ordained. For the purposes of this chapter, however, I am going to assume otherwise and will use words such as clergy, pastor, or priest to reflect this. My reason for doing this stems from the fact that while lay visitors may be called upon to provide pastoral care in medical and rehabilitation settings, it will almost always fall to the ordained leadership in a congregation to provide care for persons with mental illness. At the same time, it is true that the vast majority of clergy do not have special training in this area. Indeed, they may not want to do significant work with people who are mentally ill. This chapter is intended to be a primer for them, so they can recognize when it may be appropriate to suggest a youth or family seek more sophisticated help and to provide some means of making God's love for troubled children and youth known to them in the setting of a congregation.

One pastoral implication of mental illness is that the clergy in a congregation may be less aware that a child or youth is suffering. There are usually no obvious physical changes, and the youth simply are not hospitalized for an extended period. They are going about what appears to be the normal routine and may be seeing a therapist in the community. Children are being returned, rather quickly, to the same environment which led to the crisis. They may not have had the time to acquire many new tools to cope with that stress. The stigma in society about mental illness means many families may be reluctant to inform their clergy, especially if the mental illness involves a child or youth. Additionally, many families are aware that some clergy lack training in this area and are thus ill-equipped to help, even if entrusted with information about a child's condition. The potential exists to miss a great many pastoral care needs:

> Joseph was a fifteen-year-old who swallowed about fifteen assorted pills that he had found around the house. Upon coming to the emergency department, his stomach was pumped, which involves swallowing a rubber tube through which the contents of the stomach are removed, and then drinking a large glass of water mixed with charcoal. The charcoal acts to "soak up" excess drugs still in the digestive system. He was describing this not terribly pleasant experience and said, "Man, I'll never try *that* again!"

This is a "teachable moment" for pastoral visitors. I will usually challenge statements like the above by responding, "In a few days you are going to go right back home (or wherever). What are you going to do differently when you start having those feelings again?" Most teens do not have an immediate answer other than "I do not know" or "Not hurt myself, I guess," neither of which shows any genuine coping skill. If a child has been in therapy before such an event, the minister can ask the child to recall what the therapist has been working on: "When you feel like your parents are not listening to you, what did your counselor suggest that you do or say?" Another approach is to respond to statements such as, "I'll never try that again" with a comment that it appears that the child likes to do things impulsively and together look for ways the child might reflect before acting. This might include different ways of communicating with peers or adults, especially parents; new ways of dealing with impulsive behaviors; and new ways of dealing with anger feelings—a continuum from frustration to rage.

It is mistake to think of teenagers as "hormones with feet," which reduces them to being less than fully human. The role of the teenager is to take the world they have been given and break it apart. If play is the full-time work of children, taking their world apart and reassembling it is the full-time work of teens. Adults who are watching this process of having the world they have constructed being glibly dismantled and evaluated and remade by a teenager often struggle during these years. The pastoral visitor can certainly encourage teens to take the ideas and values and beliefs they have lived with and really look at them. Teens can put their beliefs back together in a new and hopefully more meaningful way. Ministers can help give them some religious words to these parts of their lives so that they can reassemble their worlds in light of their faith.

COGNITIVE THERAPY

Cognitive therapy has become increasingly common during the 1990s. If a pastor is involved in the lives of children who are seeing a therapist, chances are very good that some form of cognitive therapy will be involved. It is worth having a basic understanding of cognitive therapy's language and terms so that a pastoral caregiver can speak competently with psychiatrists and other mental health professionals. It is also worth knowing because this psychology is, in many ways, one of the friendliest forms of therapy to religion in general.

In order to change one's feelings, there are two options. First, one can do something to one's body, such as deep-breathing exercises. Second, one can work at changing thoughts by such means as visual images or use of words. As humans, we do not have control over anything else that will lead to different feelings. It is worth pausing here to emphasize where religion integrates very easily. Bodily changes that lead to new feelings can be brought about by certain forms of prayer styles, such as those outlined in Chapter 4. A number of studies published in medical journals document the effects of deep breathing, relaxation responses, and even prayer, which lead to lower blood pressure, lower reported stress, and lower levels of depression. The use of imagery or words in prayer that lead to changed feelings can also mesh very easily with one's religious beliefs. Again, previous examples such as icons, statues of saints, even a candle flame, or a phrase such as, "God created me and thinks that I am good" are easily integrated into one's care. It is unlikely that a therapist would suggest such religious objects or sayings. However, a pastoral caregiver with some knowledge of the child and cognitive therapy will be in an excellent position to provide pastoral care, which dovetails very neatly with other messages the child hears.

Cognitive therapy is based on the idea that each of us has had a past experience that shaped what we believe about ourselves, other people, or life in general. These beliefs will have consequences in that they will shape how we feel about new events or people and how we respond to them. Rather than delve deeply into children's feelings, cognitive therapy goes directly to the *beliefs* that influence them. The focus is on helping people identify those beliefs and working toward changing them.

Such beliefs are very often revealed by the kinds of quick-response thoughts that happen automatically when people confront a new situation or person. For example, I did some of my chaplaincy training on a particular unit that, unknown to me, had a previous bad experience with chaplains. They were not immediately accepting of me and would not speak to me when I was on the floor. My next career move took me to a hospital where there had been no chaplains before. While I was still in my first weeks, I was passed in the hall by several people in quick succession who neither responded to my "Hello!" nor made eye contact with me. The automatic thought that flashed through my mind was, "Oh, no . . . they do not like chaplains here, either. Here we go again." The reality was that I was so new at that point no one knew me. I certainly did not know the people nor the hospital culture well enough to make such a global statement about their response to chaplains. In fact, as the first chaplain in that place, many people were extremely glad for the presence of a chaplain. Automatic thoughts do not have to be true, based on fact, nor realistic. They may, in fact, be thoughts that are untrue (such as my example) or that express thoughts that are not permissible to speak aloud (such as, "God has abandoned me").

Cognitive therapy will seek to help children or youth identify what they believe, often helping them give voice to such automatic messages they give themselves. Having done that, the next step is to sort out which ones are true and which help a person function well. The others, which are not true, or which keep me from functioning as a basically happy person, are open to change. The final step is for the child to choose to change those beliefs. It takes a great deal of emotional work to reach this step, but choosing to change what one believes is not something a youth will do overnight. People of all ages frequently cling to beliefs and behaviors that are not in their best interest. Pastoral support during this process and affirmation for the work undertaken will provide new and positive experiences for the children, which can help them form new beliefs about the church, God, and themselves.

DEPRESSION

Depression is a common reason for a teenager to be involved with psychiatric care. It is important to understand what depression is *not*. All persons experience what psychiatrists call normal depressive moodswings, which are short-lived periods in which persons have sad or sullen appearance and usually prefer to be alone. Major depression is not the blues, or feeling down, nor is it short-lived. Depression is a pervasive sense of worthlessness and hopelessness that a person feels. Depression is sometimes said to be what happens when feelings of anger have no acceptable outlet and are turned inward. Teenagers typically have moodswings and may be down for several days because it can be difficult to cope with all of the changes they are going through. This is not what depression looks like. Unlike such temporary emotional low points, depression will steadily worsen without intervention. Major depression is the name given when symptoms appear for more than two weeks. This problem is not always obvious, and it is worth the pastor's time to become acquainted with the symptoms. In this way you will be in a better position to ask questions and gently suggest some additional help when it seems warranted.

The symptoms of major depression are such that pastors and parents may not suspect depression is the problem. A parent whose young child was diagnosed with depression offered two images to describe the symptoms of depression—turtles and dragons (Dubuque, 1996). Turtles, when stressed, pull their head and legs up into themselves and become quiet and stationary. Young girls with depression often act their symptoms out in a similar fashion. They become quiet, withdrawn. It might be considered just being shy. Such children rarely cause trouble at school. They are often considered "good kids" who are just reserved, and no one suspects they are depressed.

Dragons, on the other hand, are frequently noticed. They act out with dramatic displays, often with anger and outbursts of energy. Young boys frequently show dragon behavior. Their behavior does make people suspect that something is going on, but depression is not the first thing that is considered. These two images are vivid and easy to remember when thinking of a child in the congregation, but do not push them too far. No image or generalization can describe the wide variety of ways depression manifests itself, given the uniqueness of any one child. Some boys show turtle behavior and become quiet and withdrawn. Like girls, they tend to be overlooked because they are not a behavior problem. The value of these images lies in helping pastors stop and wonder what might be going on with a child who seems to fit one of these images.

Most adults who have depression appear sad or sullen; in children, depression is more likely to manifest itself in irritability. Teenagers are often sarcastic or contrary with adults, and it is easy to mistake what is going on for adolescent contrariness rather than one sign of potential depression. The symptoms may well come up more frequently in conversation with the teen or the parents. Insomnia is another symptom to be aware of, but this is not difficulty falling asleep initially. What makes the insomnia of depression noticeable is that the teen will wake up in the early morning hours (2-3 a.m.) and have difficulty going back to sleep. If you suspect that teenagers may suffer from depression, ask them how they are sleeping. If they talk about waking up in the middle of the night or very early in the morning, then let your suspicion deepen. Other symptoms include a significant change (increase or decrease) in body weight; lack of interest in activities or people that were previously very important; difficulty thinking or concentrating. Parental complaints about grades that have recently gone down can be a clue for pastors to ask about some of these other symptoms with open-ended questions that begin, "I wonder if you have seen . . ."

When several of these symptoms are seen or described, then it would be appropriate to suggest that the youth may, in fact, have a treatable condition known as depression and that a call to a physician would be a positive step to take. It is not necessary at this juncture to call a psychiatrist; whatever medical professional the youth is accustomed to seeing would be a good choice simply because that person is a familiar face. No one enjoys depression; at a deep level youth will want help even though they may resist efforts to help them.

Increasing knowledge indicates that depression has its roots in a chemical imbalance in the brain's chemistry. At the same time, many teens have limited experience in expressing, or lack the words to express, their feelings; some have learned that it is not acceptable to express them. If a physician determines that a youth genuinely has major depression, chances are good that the treatment will involve a combination of medication and some form of "talk therapy."

Most teenagers with depression do well with their treatment. The greatest danger is that once they begin to feel again, they frequently decide that the medication they have been given is no longer needed and stop taking it. Without its benefits, they may begin to slide down into past patterns of feeling and thinking. Clergy can casually ask teenagers who seem to be doing all right how things are going and remind them that it is important to use the medications.

Teenagers with depression frequently have difficulty identifying and expressing their emotions. Pastoral care of youth in a congregation can be a means to looking at and discussing biblical passages that deal with expressing feelings. An example in small group format would be to read aloud the passage of Jesus turning over the tables in the Temple (John 2:13-17) or God's anger at sinful humanity and God's decision to send the flood (Genesis 6:9-9:17). The leader can begin by asking the group to identify all of the emotions they can see described in the passage. Then the group can be asked which character experienced the feeling, what the circumstances were, and, finally, what the consequences were. Then the group can be asked if and when they have ever experienced the same feeling and what the circumstances and consequences were. With a flip-chart or whiteboard, all of the foregoing can be put into columns. The group can then be asked what similarities and differences they notice between the biblical expression of feelings and their own. The group's facilitator should be particularly watchful for youths' experiences that are overreactions to events or for feelings experienced but not expressed, and the group's facilitator should help the group name these situations. Facilitators may want to be especially ready to talk about the difference between assertive, aggressive, or passive responses to situations. In general, emotionally healthy youth are aware of and practice reasonably assertive behavior; anything that promotes this is a step toward being nurturing whole individuals.

The scriptural passages cited both deal with anger. Some other possibilities include:

- Recognizing God's gifts to us   John 4:1-26
- Goodness of created beings   Gen 1:1-31
- Grief, death, and loss   Psalm 6; Isaiah 25:6-9;
                                     Wisdom 3:1-5,9; 1 John
                                     3:1-2
- Feeling overwhelmed   Psalm 69
- "Why?"   Habakkuk, Psalm 73,
                                     John 9, Job
- Second chances   Gen 9:1-7
- Blasphemy and forgiveness   Matthew 12:31-32

It is possible for pastoral caregivers very quickly to find themselves beyond their levels of expertise and comfort. Whatever healing work pastoral caregivers have to offer will be completely overpowered by the (often unspoken) messages the children have received from their families for so many years. These situations arise no matter what level of care is offered from a congregation. Recognition of a problem may be the very best care that can be offered, at least in the beginning. The good news is that if a child has depression, it is frequently very treatable. In some cases, the child's depression or behavioral outbursts are just the most outward signs of deep-seated family problems. Such problems are frequently presented to the pastor by a parent who says to me, "Just talk with Katherine and see if you can get her to change . . ."; in a shorter form, "Fix my child." The unspoken message is, of course, that there is nothing wrong with the rest of the family. Reality is otherwise in these cases, and the situation may be felt to be so hopeless that the youth will turn toward self-injurious behaviors, which can include eraser burns, cutting on one's self with a knife or scissors, or suicide.

Some warning signs to be aware of include a recent positive moodswing after having been depressed for an extended period; the giving away of gifts or treasured possessions to others; and the more obvious verbal indications that they are thinking about harming themselves. If a clergyperson suspects a youth may be thinking about self-injurious behaviors, several steps need to be taken.

The first is to check out the suspicion and ask, "Are you thinking of hurting yourself?" If you think the youth intends suicide as opposed to lesser forms of self-harm, then ask even more specifically, "Are you thinking of taking your life?" Asking this question will not cause the youth to consider suicide, nor will it push the youth toward it if suicide has not been contemplated already. In short, *one has nothing to lose by asking this question!* The follow-up question to a positive response is to ask about a plan: "Have you thought about how you might hurt yourself?" A positive answer here is something to take quite seriously. A detailed plan indicates a serious possibility of suicide. This should always be followed by a question that examines whether the youth has the means at hand to carry out the plan: "Do you have the pills (or a knife, or whatever)?" A positive answer to both having a plan and having the means to carry it out is a threat to be taken seriously. At this point one can explain, "As your pastor, I am very concerned that you may hurt yourself, and I want very much to keep you safe. I would like to drive you to the hospital so that you can talk about this with some other people," and then go there without leaving the youth alone *even for a moment.* If you are on the phone with the youth, ask someone else to call 911 or other emergency services.

The pastor will have to adjust the wording to suit the situation and the child. Especially with middle-school-age children, it is very necessary to ask specific, concrete questions. "Are you thinking of killing yourself?" may bring an honest negative answer, but it does not reveal anything about the intentions of self-harm short of suicide. Unlike a pastoral conversation in which one asks open-ended, nonfactual questions, situations such as these require direct, closed, factual questions.

Having a detailed plan, but not the means already in one's possession, is less serious and does not require immediate action on the pastor's part, but it should certainly be followed up. An option to suggest is that the youth make a covenant for safety with you. This does not need to be an elaborate document; it can be a handwritten statement that reads:

> I, _____, agree that for the next 24 hours, until _____o'clock on _____ I will not harm myself in any way. I promise that if I feel that I want to hurt myself, I will contact Pastor _____ by telephone at _____ or come to his/her house or church at _____ and talk about my feelings. Signed, _____ and Pastor _____.

The essential elements here are a short, clearly defined time span and the willingness on the pastor's part to respond at any time during this period to the call from the youth. It is highly desirable, even if you are having this discussion on the phone, to have the youth sign the covenant. If the youth agrees to it verbally, offer to write it down and deliver it for a signature. Before the covenant expires, the pastor should contact the youth and ask how he or she is feeling at that point. If the youth indicates no feelings about self-harm, then the pastor can let go and perhaps make a phone call in another twenty-four hours. If feelings of ambivalence or strong inclinations toward self-harm are still present, another covenant can be written and signed and the process repeated, or one might suggest that the situation is serious enough that the pastor would like to take the youth to a hospital to talk about his or her feelings with another professional. In the morning hours, many youth will have some hope for the day. By midafternoon, they are more likely to feel that they just cannot take it anymore; this is perhaps the most difficult part of the day. Pastors wishing to check up on a teenager they are concerned about may want to time their calls or visits with this in mind. It is also necessary for the pastor to inform another responsible adult that this contract for safety has been signed. Other responsible adults include the parents or guardians or the child's therapist. If a pastoral caregiver has a youth sign such a contract and then fails to inform another adult responsible for the child's well-being, that pastoral caregiver is liable should any harm come to the child.

> Marjorie is a lay pastoral visitor with some training and is from a mainline Protestant congregation. A female, adolescent church member was hospitalized following a suicide attempt by swallowing many different pills. Visiting the teen on the medical floor, Marjorie began her conversation by exclaiming, "Why would a pretty girl like you try to kill herself?"

This pastoral visit got off to a false start and did not cover any real substantial ground. Later, Marjorie was trying to understand what might have improved her visit. She forgot that meaningful pastoral care involves the awareness of how one's personal values can get in the way. Marjorie's presupposition was that physically attractive adolescent women have no logical reason to experience a sense of hopelessness or worthlessness. Of course, there is no need to check your own beliefs at the door. One the other hand, the pastoral caregiver must be aware of how a person's own thoughts and feelings can block effective listening. This is especially true when visiting teenagers who have tried to hurt themselves. In many cases, being judged is precisely what they are afraid God is doing. To some degree, the pastor has an opportunity to negate that sense of painful reproach.

Teenagers' feelings of judgment may, in fact, be a good place to begin a conversation (and certainly better than beginning by asking them "Why?" they have done something). In my experience, teenagers who have engaged in self-injurious behaviors are concerned with their relationship with God. They ask: Have I committed the unpardonable sin? Will God punish me for this? Why did God let this happen to me?

The spectrum of answers to those questions is broad. In discussing this topic with a number of clergy, having time to engage in theological reflection alone or with a few peers in the context of a congregational clergy's job is considered a luxury. Nevertheless, take some time to consider how you would answer the teenagers' questions about God and suicide, or attempted suicide. How do you explain or define the "unpardonable sin"? For what actions does God punish humanity? How involved do you believe God is in the minute acts of life? Does God step in to cause or prevent events in daily life—and how was God active in an event such as this?

In a Spiritual Issues Group on a hospital psychiatric unit, I was initially surprised by the level of interest in the end of the world. A working knowledge of the apocalyptic literature in the Bible is very, very helpful in understanding where their ideas are coming from. Someone who makes frequent reference to these passages may also voice a sense that we are already living in the end times. In such cases, living in the end times may be taken as a license or rationalization for behavior. It is a mistake, I believe, to allow the Scriptures to be abused as a crutch or a rationalization for unhealthy behavior. For example, someone should not use references to the book of Revelation about the end times to justify an attitude that any behavior is permissible.

If you observe this situation, you may invite the youth into an extended conversation, one that will probably need to occur over a longer period of time than a single visit affords. To do that, the pastor first needs to break down the youth's statements into their root issues in order to identify and get to the religious issues. These religious issues may then be examined one at a time. To take the second example from the previous paragraph that "it does not matter," you can identify to yourself the various levels that are involved. There is a sense of hopelessness about both present and future and a sense of powerlessness in the youth's ability to change the situation for the better. This latter spiritual issue suggests low self-esteem, which in turn suggests that the youth has difficulty appreciating his or her status as a child of God. It is this breakdown of the psychiatric problem into religious language that is the pastoral visitor's specialty and calling.

For example, consider the following conversation between a chaplain and two teenagers, Rich and Suzy:

> **Rich** (rolls up his sleeve to show where he has cut on himself): This is what God has done—nothing! Why would God let this go on?

> **Suzy:** Yeah, I mean, we are on our own. It says in the Bible that we are damned because we tried to kill ourselves, right? So why does anything matter?

Chaplain: You feel that God has abandoned you because God did not step in to protect you?

Rich: You got it!

Chaplain: Sounds pretty dismal and lonely. I wonder, what would make life look better?

Suzy: (pause) Nothing.

Rich: Maybe being dead, but we will probably burn, so that is no better than here.

The conversation continues for a while and then ends with the following:

Chaplain: If you had to come up with a name for this group, what would you choose?

Rich: Vomit of the gods!

The two youths depicted express a sense of hopelessness. God has not left them to fend for themselves and has not come to rescue them from their situation. Nor is there any expectation for life to improve; neither person is able to identify concrete actions or events that they would regard as better. The passive acceptance of their fate (". . . we are damned . . .") and the group name Rich created reflect their low self-esteem. Suzy regards Scripture as condemning her, neglecting Scripture's almost implicit *approval* of Samson's suicide (Judges 16:30). Although brief, this conversation is ripe with possible starting points for further discussion. Here a clergyperson can make a unique contribution to the child's healing. Although they are being treated by other professionals for depression and self-injurious behavior, no one else will approach the issues of self-esteem, guilt, and self-condemnation from the perspective of being God's child and God's good gift! In addition to using this language with the youth, the ability to interpret religious issues in terms of the emotions which accompany them gives the pastor the ability to converse in meaningful ways with counselors and psychiatrists.

The first time you sit down with teenagers to walk through these issues should not be the first time you have ever tried to put these ideas into words. Provide them with an emotionally safe spot to raise the questions, and demonstrate that they are worth listening to and that you value what they have to say. This may be at least as important as any theological response. The pastoral response to these youth is the one that invites them to share their questions about God. And, questions about God they certainly do have.

EATING DISORDERS

Being outside the family circle and yet having frequent contact with youth, clergy are in an excellent position to take note of changes they see. Depression is one mental health condition that clergy might identify and name to the youth or parents. Another condition is an eating disorder. Eating disorders include anorexia nervosa, in which a person uses extreme means to lower one's weight based on a false image of one's own body, and bulimia, in which a person will binge and then purge the food from one's system in an attempt to control body size. This, too, is based on a distorted sense of self. Between 90 and 95 percent of anorexics are female. It is important to understand that body size, eating, and food are simply the grounds on which a much larger battle is being waged. They are the *means* and not the end.

At their root, eating disorders are about *control.* Teenagers with eating disorders use food to cope with, or have some control over, a variety of adolescent issues. These may include identity; low self-esteem; conflicting feelings about one's family; their emerging adult bodies and sexuality; and sometimes child abuse. Although most adolescents with an eating disorder will initially claim to have developed purging habits because they think they are overweight, at the primary level, their unhealthy behaviors provide them with one facet of life that they can control.

As with teenagers who have depression, many who have eating disorders also have difficulty talking about their feelings. This might not be suspected from the typical profile of someone who suffers from anorexia or bulimia. To the extent that a "typical" profile exists, it would be an adolescent female; usually a high achiever in school and frequently an honor student; someone highly articulate; one who frequently displays "all or nothing" thinking; and frequently one who is the daughter of a very controlling and/or perfectionistic father.

Naturally, not all thin, intelligent, adolescent females should be viewed as candidates for this disease. When a clergyperson is aware of other warning signs, it may well be time to take some action. These signs include noticeable weight loss; complaints about feeling fat when, in fact, the body size is appropriate or even on the thin side; denying hunger at a time when her peers are eating (such as a youth group event) or eating very small amounts of food; or spending a significant amount of time alone, or preferring to eat alone. An extreme sign is when a youth who is a member of a eucharistic church refuses even the elements of bread and wine at communion.

A good first step is to check out one's suspicions with the youth's mother or father by sharing one's fears and noting how the warning signs seem to be present. One might also share those concerns with the girl's family physician. This is a case where speaking directly to the youth may not be very productive. Similar to substance abusers or addicts, adolescents with an eating disorder are extremely clever at denying or hiding their disease process. Nevertheless, an expression of concern for her health and safety can be made, and the youth should be encouraged to make a visit to the doctor.

Pastoral care of youth will involve more than simply encouraging one to turn his or her life over to God. The values and thoughts of someone with anorexia or bulimia have parallels in the early gnostic heresy, with its denial of the body as a good thing. The thinking of those with anorexia is so distorted that they have moved beyond "my body is not what I want" to "my body is bad." Since the psychological root of eating disorders is the control that they afford youth, this is also a good place to begin from a pastoral perspective. Control is a psychological concept, and it is also a religious concept. One way to think about eating disorders is that they provide control over self, and exaltation of that control has become a god. The disease becomes almost idolatrous, in that it dictates one's values, thoughts, and actions. For the pastoral visitor who has or who can build a trusting relationship with a teen suffering from an eating disorder, the pastor can introduce biblical passages, such as the creation narratives in Genesis, which affirm creation as God's and as inherently good. Naturally, one cannot simply point to these and expect the youth to assent to them. On the other hand, one might begin by reading the story aloud with the youth and ask open, reflective questions such as, "How does this compare with the way you see God?" or "What is it like to have God call your body 'good'?"

Questions that invite them to talk about their relationship with God or how close they feel to God are also helpful. In my experience, many of the teenage girls who have eating disorders share a perspective in common with those who make suicidal gestures. That is, they feel that because of their self-injurious actions, God has or will condemn them. They feel distant and judged by God. A perspective I have heard that is unique is that they *personalize* responsibility for their actions. They feel that their actions have *hurt* God; that God is suffering and sorry for what they have done. This is a grandiose statement: I have the power to hurt God. At the same time, they can verbalize that they see God demonstrating anger, wrath, aching, yearning, and joy as a result of what God's creatures do. I suggest not being distracted by the grandiosity and using this as a starting point to discuss other ways to influence God. What changes do you think you can make that would make God rejoice? How might you seek God's forgiveness for the hurt? This latter might be prefaced by asking how she goes about seeking forgiveness after hurting someone she knows well.

IDENTITY AND SELF-ESTEEM ISSUES

Tania typifies a more commonly encountered pastoral need:

Tania is a sixteen-year-old and a hard-working student who began to go to church with her grandparents about three years ago, largely because of the restaurant brunch that followed mass. When she was approached about making her first communion last year, she enthusiastically began the preparation and found it to be a high point of her life. A year later, she now feels distant from a God whom she views as punishing her, evidenced by something bad happening after every good event. "What happened that I went from being really into God, to this?" When asked what she would like to hear God tell her today, she replies, "That my disease is not me and that He is always here for me."

Tania is a typical teenager. She is experiencing the normal ups and downs of adolescence—in one week she won a medal at a statewide academic contest, and she learned of a grandparent's diagnosis of a terminal illness. Holding such emotionally laden events in her mind at the same time was difficult, and her questions in the vignette express that struggle.

In psychological terms, Tania's sense of distance from God and her sense that God is sending bad things her way have taught her that she deserves them. She believes that she is not worth God's time to go after and rescue; what she wants to hear so desperately is that she is worthy of God's love. If this were to continue, it is not difficult to envision how a teenager's sense of self-worth would diminish. And this during the years when self-worth is a fragile thing to begin with.

A pastoral caregiver might diagnose a spiritual issue and approach the teen from two angles. At present, Tania has an overwhelmingly transcendent image of God as powerful (able to send bad events her way after every good one) and as a judge (who sentences her to punishment). This perception of God may lead her to lack an appreciation of herself as one of God's own creatures whom God loves. Experiences of an immanent God, one who is near at hand and personal, provides a first balance to the spiritual problem of feeling distant from God. Biblical images abound where God has been close to, and even social with, humanity. The three visitors to Abraham and Sarah (Genesis 18) bring momentous news in a most unassuming way: as travelers over a meal thrown together at the last minute. Resurrection appearances of Jesus along the Emmaus road and over a fish breakfast on the water's edge (John 21) are similar examples.

One might invite a youth to recall a time when a friend or a family member dropped by unexpectedly. What was that like? Did he or she enjoy the visit? Did he or she feel connected to a larger group, such as their circle of friends or extended family, even though he or she could not see the entire group at the time? That which connects us to a community connects us to God at some level. If the teenager is old enough to have had a boyfriend or girlfriend, the pastoral caregiver might invite a recollection of the feelings for that person and suggest that God has strong feelings for us and wants to love us. The glimpse of the Divine that loving relationships give to us can be held up by pastors as reminders of God—something teens and adults alike forget all too easily.

A discussion along these lines might be with an individual or with an entire youth group or class with contributions from everyone's experience. Journaling is an option a pastor might suggest to a teenager feeling distant, with the twist that the journal be a letter to God. The letter might include anything from describing the events of one's day to asking God for a concrete message, such as answering the question put to Tania in the vignette: "What would you like to hear God tell you today?"

The second approach is to use images that affirm the worth and dignity of every person. The creation story in Genesis, culminating in the pronouncement of creation as good, is an obvious choice. There is a useful distinction to be made between goodness and holiness. Creation and humanity are good but not necessarily holy. We are good in God's eyes, but we are not perfect, nor are we expected to be. Making mistakes, doing things we later regret, even letting our relationship with God grow distant are all very human predicaments. Teens striving to be perfect and to meet the conflicting demands and pressures of family, peers, school, and congregation may need to be given permission to cut themselves some slack! Paul's letter to the Romans (5:8) is another passage that affirms our value and worth to God, even though we are less-than-perfect sinners.

Pastoral care that builds relationships with children and youth, and begins early, before there is a crisis of any kind, goes a long way toward the formation of a healthy people. The affirmation, in explicitly religious terms, of the worth and dignity of every child, youth, and adult is an expression of God's love and concern, which will enable them to deal with life's crises from a stronger vantage point.

CONFIDENTIALITY ISSUES

Pastoral caregivers find themselves moving through an incredible variety of situations. By the very nature of the ministry, they quickly become privy to an immense amount of story that has been told to them. Being taken into the confidence of so many people, and to such a depth, often has an awe-inspiring effect, and one holds those stories as sacred gifts. There are times, however, where simply holding on to someone's story may not be in anyone's best interest. The issue of confidentiality is a difficult one because few, if any, religious traditions have any guidelines for what may be openly discussed. The few that exist are general rubrics governing rites of reconciliation (more commonly called confession) and state that the priest is under the absolute moral obligation to maintain the secrecy of that conversation. Beyond that, there is little official guidance.

This becomes problematic for the pastor seriously interested in providing pastoral care as part of a network of professionals working for the benefit of the child because most, if not all, of the other professionals have such guidelines. Psychiatrists and therapists are often unable to acknowledge that a particular child is, in fact, a patient, much less be willing to share or listen to information. Their trust level for clergy is sometimes low because clergy are perceived as being too ready to share information and as having no professional standards to which they are accountable. Acknowledging this and stating that one intends to be very respectful of confidentiality will begin to forge a trusting relationship with other professionals. In general, psychiatrists and therapists will need a written release signed by the parent before they will work with you. You may want to approach the parents about writing and signing such a release, and ask that they deliver it to the person you would like to make contact with. Some of the mistrust also arises from other professionals' perceptions that clergy too readily enter into relationships and or topics that are "over their heads" and then find themselves unable to give any real help to the child. In your initial contact, you might outline the kind of care you envision providing and how that relates to the work of others.

Confidentiality is confusing because of the nature of how pastors acquire information and stories. In the course of a single conversation, one may be taken to different levels of intimacy by a youth. Or one might overhear information while attending a youth group event. Does that merit the same protection as information a teen might relate to you in the hospital? The question becomes one of what and how much is the pastor free to discuss with others, or even how much to bring up with the person again. From the layperson's perspective, much, if not all, of what is related to the pastoral caregiver (ordained or not) is secret. It is assumed it will go no further.

Some professionals have distinguished a hierarchical system of increasing obligations to maintain pastoral information as completely private. The Association of Professional Chaplains has adopted a more conservative position in their Code of Ethics, which regards virtually all information as confidential. Such information may only be shared on rare occasions, "for the enhancement of the health and well-being of an individual or when required by law" (Association of Professional Chaplains). This is more in line with what youth will expect of the pastor, and it is the safest way to go. The person who has told you part of a story must give you permission to relate the story to another individual. Those persons should also understand that the information is to go no farther. The exception to this would be when someone is in danger. Consider the following example:

> Janna was a sixteen-year-old girl who was raped by her date one night. Her pastor visited her at the hospital and offered to have her included in the prayer chain of the congregation. Janna gave her permission for the pastor to share her story with the prayer chain so that they could make their prayers specific to her needs. Members of the prayer chain, however, told other members of the congregation, and people began to make comments to Janna's family members and inquired about her condition. The rape had caused Janna to cease being able to trust people; the knowledge that "the whole church knows" simply made an awful situation more difficult for her.

There are times when it may benefit someone for the pastoral caregiver to tell what is known about the child or youth. Anyone to whom information is given, however, should be given some guidance about whether such information is to be held in confidence or if it may be shared. Prayer chains have tremendous value; even children and teens talk about feeling supported in their healing knowing that the prayer chain of a congregation is praying for them. The weak point in a prayer chain is the extent to which it understands and observes confidentiality in how it operates. Breaking confidentiality, as the example above demonstrates, creates additional pain for people.

What children or youth say to you, they should be able to say with the expectation that you will not share such information with their parents or guardians. One of the fundamental premises of this book is that you are the child's pastor, and your relationship with that child or youth is every bit as important as your relationship with any adult in the congregation. One implication of this is that the same rules apply to your relationship with children and teenagers as to your relationship with adults. It may be worthwhile reminding children and youth of this as they may feel more free to say what is really on their minds or ask a question without fear of being judged by their parents. At the same time, parents may ask you about conversations you have had with their child, and you may need to remind them of the boundaries of your relationship.

Chapter 6

A Theological Reflection

"Why did God take my child, Pastor? She never had a chance to live out her life. Why can she not have lived until she was eighty? How could God do that?" The pastor spread his hands, and said, "I do not know."

A pastor notices during the worship services that one of the teenage acolytes seems to be on the verge of tears. After the service she is being comforted by several other adolescents. Inquiring of the teen's mother if she knows of anything that is amiss, she relates that a classmate of her daughter's, who also used to be her daughter's boyfriend, committed suicide the previous day. As the pastor approaches, the teen turns to the pastor and sobs, "Why didn't God stop him? How could God let this happen?" And the teens who were with her all looked at the pastor with expectant faces, waiting for his answer.

Perhaps no event in earthly life can bring out the agonizing cry of "Why, O God?" like the dying and death of a child. The sense of helplessness that pastoral caregivers can feel when confronted with these questions can be awesome and even paralyzing. As I noted in the beginning of this book, a midcareer, highly successful congregational pastor who has never experienced the death of a child in a congregation he has served feels that he is "living on borrowed time" before he is confronted with these questions. The fear stems in part from the sense of inadequacy of any answer in the face of such an ultimate question. The fear is also a natural fear of the unknown. Most clergy who have never faced these questions from an anguished parent or teenager have never given a great deal of thought to what they might say nor given much reflective thought to how they approach pastoral care.

I strongly advocate thinking these issues through before being confronted by a child who is asking these questions or one who is actively dying. Virtually no one will ever ask you for a theological discourse on death at coffee hour or while shaking hands after a service. It is not inconceivable, however, that you might be confronted with this while making a newcomer visit, during which an old wound is reopened when the pastor inquires about a child's photograph, only to discover that the child has died and the family still grieves. The second of the opening vignettes happened to me one Sunday morning in a congregation and is another example of how this issue can suddenly arise.

RESPONSES TO THE NATURE OF SUFFERING

There is no single answer to the question of why children become gravely ill or are victims of traumatic injuries and die. The image of a jewel held up to a light is helpful: if the jewel is turned, light will reflect differently off of each facet. So it is also in dealing with the mystery that is death. Numerous attempts have been made over centuries to respond to these issues. A few approaches are outlined here, and their value is to be a resource for further reflection by pastoral caregivers. The most meaningful responses will be those that are consistent with the belief system of the parents and the child and those that are genuine and grounded in the reflections of the pastoral caregiver.

Scriptural Responses

Scripture is often cited by many pastoral caregivers as addressing questions of evil, suffering, and the nature of God, and so it does. It does not, however, speak with one voice. Nor does every part of Scripture that touches on these issues touch equally on all of them. The writers of Scripture sought to interpret their experiences in light of their beliefs. Sometimes they sought to justify God's actions; other times to hold believers accountable for the suffering that had befallen them. All of the scriptural responses to the question of suffering are a reading back of God's actions into an event—an attempt to deal with these issues looking at them from hindsight. The Book of Job is perhaps the most frequently quoted part of Scripture in addressing these questions, but there are numerous other attempts to respond to this issue. Pastoral caregivers may therefore turn to it without looking at the other resources available to them. What follows is a summary of the variety of voices with which Scripture speaks.

Psalm 37 permits suffering in the present because in the end, God will punish the evildoers: "Do not fret yourself because of evil-doers. . . . For they shall soon wither like the grass, and like the green grass fade away" (Psalm 37:1a, 2, *The Book of Common Prayer*, 1979). The day will come for the wicked, and in the mean-time, the righteous should devote themselves to following the way of the *Lord* and seeking justice. The suggestion that the righteous will enjoy the blessings of God is often taken by youth (and by adults) to assume that in the face of illness or tragedy, they have not led righteous lives. This can be a source of dismay to those who have sought to conform their lives to their beliefs, believing that right actions will always lead to a life that is free from suffering. Children whose thinking is still in a concrete stage (approximately five to ten years of age) frequently experience such dismay.

Proverbs 3:11, 12 suggests that suffering is educational, a fre-quent theme in Scripture. In particular, suffering is, or at least can be, caused by the *Lord* as a method of discipline. Suffering here is actually a sign of the *Lord's* love, for if the *Lord* did not care for the creature, the *Lord* would not bother disciplining the creature. The challenge for the pastoral caregiver is to distinguish between two ways to understand the point of suffering: on the one hand, a God who inflicts trauma to teach humans a lesson and, on the other hand, a redemptive quality that may come out of a traumatic event after someone reflects and thinks in new ways. Adults sometimes have the most difficulty comprehending a God such as this. Children, on the other hand, may find this the easiest image to relate to since they have experienced being disciplined by their parents. The fact that children may easily comprehend it does not mean it is the most helpful image to offer, however.

The pastor may be able to draw the parallel here for them, but caution should be exercised. If the children do not experience their parents as loving, then this image will serve only to confirm that God is no different and probably no better than their parents. It may suggest a God who is interested in judgment, punishment, and reproof as God's primary responses to humans rather than mercy, forgiveness, and compassion. Pastors need to draw upon their knowledge of the children's family dynamics and also their religious tradition's understanding of Scripture and God's interaction with humans before using this illustration with children and youth. For some resources on ways religion has been used to oppress others, especially children, refer to the bibliography.

The Book of Habakkuk is a seldom-quoted text that seeks to explain the apparent inequity of people who do bad deeds and get away with them while the righteous suffer. One difference is that this book is concerned with suffering on a national scale. Israel is being threatened by the Chaldeans because of their own iniquity. Some suffering, at least, is deserved. Some pastoral caregivers are quick to hold up their hands and dismiss all suffering as not being understandable; this book places the cause squarely on the sufferers. The suffering they will undergo is not to be permanent, nor will any evil power gain a permanent upper hand. The response that is worked out through the prophet's vision is more well-known: wait and endure patiently now because, in the end, the *Lord* will make everything right.

No biblical resource is more used than the story of Job. Job is the most fully developed attempt to work through the issue of suffering and unjust events. There are five clear answers to the issue of evil befalling one of God's children, each answer taken up by one or more characters. The first of these is the idea that suffering occurs as a test of a believer. This is seen most clearly in the first two chapters of the book in the dialogue between God and the satan. This is also the Islamic response to suffering. Legitimate questions that may be posed to persons who view their experiences in this way would be, "Are you passing?" or "How can I help you succeed?"

The concept of Divine Retribution, in which God punishes sinners because of their sins, is the position given voice by the three "friends" who come to visit Job. This has some parallels on an individual scale with the response given in the book of Habakkuk on a national scale. A difference, though, is that suffering in Divine Retribution will only cease when one repents and changes one's way of living.

The third response from the Book of Job is the idea that at least some suffering is educational. The character Elihu makes this point in Chapters 32 to 37. This is similar to the portion of Proverbs cited earlier.

The fourth response is that of Job himself, which he puts forth in various places throughout the text. He argues that there is no reason. Suffering is completely devoid of meaning, something which simply must be endured.

The final response, put forth by the voice of the *Lord* speaking out of the whirlwind, is that suffering is a mystery (Chapters 38 to 42:6). Only this last response to the questions posed by Job is allowed to stand by the author. In fact, the author proceeds to show God's wrath rising up against the four men who spoke with Job. There are many occasions when silence before a mystery is an excellent pastoral response. Many people find nothing is more mysterious and difficult to comprehend than why suffering or other difficult events involve children. There are times when the best pastoral care is hesitant to rush in with answers or, indeed, with any words. I would include miscarriages, stillbirths, and unexplained infant deaths such as those from sudden infant death syndrome in this category.

The idea that suffering provides an opportunity to demonstrate the divine power of God's activity came when the Christian church weighed in with its response in the story of Jesus' interaction with the man born blind and his parents (John 9). The disciples' starting point is the same as the first three of Job's visitors: they subscribe to the idea of Divine Retribution and assume that the suffering this man endures because of his blindness is the result of someone's action. The only question for them is whose: the man's or his parents'? Jesus answers the question to make the point that the cause is immaterial, but something redemptive can come out of his experience. That something is people seeing God at work in healing and people responding to this by giving glory to God. Jesus ignores the "Why?" question in favor of pointing to God's work in the world. Suffering exists, but the more fundamental question for Jesus is the human response to it.

Paul echoes this idea in his letter to the Romans (5:1-5) in which he links the experience of suffering with its shape on one's character. Any experience with suffering must change a person. The question is: how will it change us? Neither this passage nor the one from John would be very appropriate to offer in the midst of a pastoral crisis. Having walked through the valley and come out the other side with a child or parent, both of these passages offer a starting point to sit down and look at what effect it has had. "I am wondering what is different for you?" "I am wondering how life is different for you after this experience?" Open-ended questions such as this provide a starting point for helping children and youth talk about what impact an event has had on their lives.

Two Contemporary Responses

The twentieth century has produced numerous works that address the question of suffering (some of these are cited in the annotated bibliography at the end of this book). Many pastoral caregivers will be familiar with the more popular books available today, and seminary-trained persons have likely been exposed to academic theological writings on this issue. This is not all that can be said on the topic, however. Two significant works are little known to American pastoral caregivers, yet they make a valuable contribution to the discussion of suffering and its meaning. Both of these were born out of tragedy and of trying to read meaning back into the event. The first event is the bombing of London during World War II and an English clergyman's attempt to deal with the issue from the pulpit. The second is a father's attempt to discover meaning and God following the death of his twenty-one-year-old son while mountain climbing in Switzerland.

We use the phrase God's will to describe so many events in human life, both happy and tragic. That the phrase is used so loosely is hardly new. Leslie Weatherhead was the preacher at the City Temple, a London congregation, during World War II. In an attempt to help them understand, in terms of their faith, the bombing they were undergoing, he preached a series of sermons about the will of God. These were subsequently published. Weatherhead attacked the issue of what is God's will for humanity, and how we discern it, quite directly.

He begins by noting how widely used the term God's will is— such that it was in danger of having little or no meaning (Weatherhead, 1944). For his purposes, he differentiates the will of God into three categories. The first he calls God's intentional will. This is God's dream for each person growing into fullness. Were there no evil or sin in the world, God's intentional will is all that we would see. It is what God intended from the very beginning in the Garden and what He intends for each of us throughout our lives. Weatherhead would also argue, I think, that God's intentional will exists for whole communities, such as the church or all Americans, just as the will exists on an individual level.

The reality of human life is, however, not Garden-like. Evil and sin and even simple carelessness abound. When circumstances occur that frustrate or even temporarily contradict God's intentional will, God still has a preference for us among the choices that confront us. Weatherhead calls this God's circumstantial will, known colloquially as the lesser of two evils. The prime example for Weatherhead is the crucifixion of Jesus. God did not intend for Jesus to call all persons to God through this instrument of death and torture. The intentional, ideal will was for all persons to follow Jesus based on what they saw and heard. This is not what happened. Given the sinful ways in which humanity responded to Jesus and his message, Jesus was confronted with several options. He could summon all godly power and bring in the new kingdom violently, or he could submit to death on the cross and use it to call others to the sacrificial love he had sought to model throughout his life. He could have, perhaps, run and hidden away in the wilderness until an opportune moment when people might better hear his news. Having such choices before him, Jesus discerned that, in this case, the option of crucifixion was closest to what he had been preaching about for three years. In that sense, and that sense only, the cross was, indeed, God's will. The death of children, whether through sudden infant death syndrome or cancer, is not what God intends for them. In these circumstances, it is not God's will to alter the laws of nature to permit these children to live, nor to intervene and will human belief in God through a dramatic act.

Weatherhead defines a third category, which he calls God's ulti-mate will. This is his way of saying that nothing finally will defeat God's intentional will from being carried out. It may take a long time, and it may only be visible when we have a different perspec-tive, but God's dreams for humanity will finally be realized. Al-though his book was published before the end of the war, this event is a good illustration of his categories. God intends for humans to live in peace and in world community with one another. Circum-stances arise, however, due to corporate sin or evil, that permit persons such as Hitler, Stalin, and Pol Pot to rise to oppressive power. In that case, Weatherhead contends, it is God's circumstan-tial will to put them down, even though this means death for the cream of a society's young people. The defeat of such people and the restoration of peace shows that God's ultimate will does indeed prevail, although it may be seen only through a horrible meantime.

One of the very great values of Weatherhead's work is that he helps us get our thinking right about our terms:

> Sonja was a three-month-old girl who was brought to the hospital emergency room after her parents discovered her not breathing in her crib. Despite all attempts to resuscitate her, she had indeed died. The parent's pastor arrived at the hospital to comfort them. Patting Sonja's head, he turned to the parents and said, "Dry your tears. This was God's will."

The phrase God's will is too easily bandied about by pastoral care-givers because it sounds pious and comforting. Indeed, many per-sons use it intending to be comforting in the face of tragedy. It is a phrase that should not be used lightly but only when one under-stands all that can be implied by it and all that it may mean to the listener. An objection to Weatherhead's work is precisely the fact that phrases about death, even the death of children, being God's will *are* comforting. Why should pastoral caregivers not use lan-guage that is a comfort to people? It seems to be the very last thing we should worry about as pastoral caregivers.

Statements such as, "It was God's will," whether made by par-ents or pastoral persons, can be comforting and, therefore, valuable because they perpetuate the myth that God is in charge, despite apparent evidence to the contrary (Allen, 1992). Pastors who spend any time at all listening to congregants will hear words such as this used to give meaning to sudden, usually tragic, events. When such language is used in the midst of chaos, such as what might have occurred in the emergency department with the infant Sonja from the previous vignette, it might be that the person using such language does not actually believe the event to be the will of God. Instead, at that moment, the words are spoken on a mythical, not a literal, level and mean that in the midst of horrible chaos, despite all the indications to the contrary, somehow God is in charge and in control of all things. These words are, in a sense, affirming the reality of God's ultimate will, to use Weatherhead's terms. There are times when events are so horrible that one must cling to the fundamental myths of our faith to express something that is too true to be spoken aloud.

Weatherhead would probably replace the word myth in Allen's usage with the word lie, or at least, untruth. He would insist that pastoral caregivers explicitly correct persons when they make such utterances, even if such words are spoken in the midst of a tragic moment in a hospital or at the graveside. The objection that I make to this is that it assumes the pastoral caregiver can look into the hearts of suffering persons and discern their beliefs. When given the opportunity to speak, parents or children will seek to communicate the meaning of their experiences in the best available language that they have in the moment. These metaphors ought to be respected by the pastoral caregiver.

The second contemporary response is contained in a slender volume written by Nicholas Wolterstorff and titled *Lament for a Son*. It is the words of a father coming to grips with the death of his young adult son who was mountain climbing in Switzerland. Reading this book is perhaps the nearest one can get, without having actually gone through that event, to understanding what a parent experiences when a child dies. The author comes to find the meaning in learning that suffering and love are inseparably linked. The love that exists between God and humans always involves suffering; the love that exists between humans, to the extent that it mirrors God's love for us, is also going to involve suffering. Without being willing to risk the hurt that comes through suffering, one never truly loves as deeply and wholly as one might.

Wolterstorff, as with others who have seen suffering closely, has a large tolerance for the presence of the mysterious. While leaving the details to the mysterious realm of God, he also finds an educational aspect to suffering. It is through suffering deeply that one learns of the giftedness of life—how utterly precious and precarious life truly is. Neither understanding life as a gift nor the linkage of suffering and love are "answers" to the question, "Why does this horrible thing happen to my child?" for this author. At the same time, he discovers no other way to have gained the new awareness without having experienced such a tragic and painful loss.

To gain this awareness, and to change one's life because of this awareness, is to share in God's own life and to show it forth to others. Wolterstorff takes quite seriously the words from the biblical book of Genesis which state that humans are created in the image of God. Our suffering is a small experience of God's suffering over Jesus' death and the continuing ways in which humanity rejects God's loving creation. Our suffering can teach us the giftedness of life, and our sense of its fragility and preciousness may affect the way we interact with and respond to others around us. Suffering is not in vain when it changes lives. The author would never suggest that his learning and suffering are equivalents, but he is able to find the redemptive out of the horrible, not unlike God.

A Personal Response

While acknowledging that no answer is perfect, over time I have developed an understanding and response to such ultimate questions of life and death, especially as they are asked about children's experiences. These responses inform how I approach pastoral care in general, and at times, I share some of this with children or their parents. I relate it here simply as a model of what I advocate all pastoral caregivers should develop for themselves. My undergraduate work in astrophysics clearly plays a role in my belief, and others may interpret scientific work differently or not regard it as having a place in theological discourse. Certainly not everyone will agree with what I have written, but I recall from one very helpful seminary professor that what I appreciated most was how his theology was so well thought out that it gave me something firm to rebel against or to adopt in some way myself. Out of my questions, the following has emerged.

Dying is part of living; for Christians it is the doorway from one life into the next. Any discussion of death and dying must necessarily begin with a discussion of living. Here, then, is an example of how I have worked out living and dying using my experience and religious tradition. All who read this book will, I hope, work out their own, and I offer the following reflection not to convince others of my position but as a model for their own work.

Humans are God's creatures, formed and made out of the dust of the earth (Genesis 2:7). The Episcopal church's burial rites include this beginning and ending in dust in the commendation of the departed: "You only are immortal, the creator and maker of mankind; and we are mortal, formed of the earth, and to earth shall we return. For so did you ordain when you created me, saying, 'You are dust, and to dust you shall return.' All of us go down to the dust; yet even at the grave, we make our song: Alleluia, alleluia, alleluia" (*Book of Common Prayer*, 1979).

What we know from Scripture and the hymns of the ancient church is also affirmed in other ways as well. One of Joni Mitchell's songs ("Woodstock," 1969) included the line "We are stardust." This is *literally* and figuratively true. The best model contemporary cosmologists have to describe scientifically what occurred at the moment of creation is commonly referred to as the "Big Bang." There was a point source that suddenly—by mechanisms the cosmologists do not attempt to describe and which theologians call God—exploded outward with immense amounts of energy. There was, in fact, so much energy that only atoms could exist. Atoms are the smallest particles of matter that can exist and still retain the properties of matter. Another way of saying that this was a high energy period is to say that the temperature was extraordinarily hot. Heat caused the atoms to move so rapidly and with such force that it was impossible for any of them to join together. The only element of matter that existed at the moment of creation was the simplest of all—hydrogen gas, which is composed simply of one single atom. If two hydrogen atoms were even to approach each other, their energy level was so great that they would bounce off each other and fly off in another direction.

As time went on, the temperature began to go down, and concentrations of hydrogen gas could begin to form small clouds. These clouds began to clump together, and eventually they would have enough mass that the gravitational pull would be so great that the cloud would collapse in upon itself. When that happened, the pressure in the middle of the cloud would increase, and the hydrogen atoms began to increase in temperature. At some point, if the cloud was big enough and had enough gravitational pull on itself, the pressure in the middle of the cloud would be so high that fusion would begin to occur. Now when two hydrogen atoms approached each other, the pressure was so great that they were slammed together and forced to be one happy molecule. Since there are two atoms, this new molecule is not hydrogen anymore, but the element helium. When nuclear fusion begins to occur, the cloud is said to become a star, such as our sun, and stars contentedly burn hydrogen into helium for most of their lives. When they deplete the supply of hydrogen, they begin to fuse helium into lithium, the next most complex molecule. Stars will later begin to burn lithium into heavier elements, all of which collect inside the star's core until it finally reaches the "iron limit," by which point the first twenty-six elements have been fused and much of them burned by the star.

Elements heavier than iron would require the addition of outside energy to create, and the only way the cosmos knows how to do that is through the death of the star. How a star dies is entirely determined by the size or mass of the initial hydrogen cloud. Stars more than three times the mass of our sun die in a fiery supernova. The energy of that stellar explosion is so great that the pressure and temperature can take the iron molecules and fuse them into heavier and heavier elements. At the same time it flings these molecules out into space where eventually they clump together and form all the matter of space. In this manner, all of the ninety-two naturally occurring elements were formed inside a star or at its spectacular death. We, the pages of this book, and the roadway on which we travel to work are all quite literally stardust.

This is the dust of creation into which God's own *ruah* is breathed to enliven it into humanity. The Hebrew word *ruah* translates equally well as wind, breath, or spirit. The *ruah* of God is the breath which animates the dust out of which humanity is created

(Genesis 2:7). Without this breath within us, we die and return to the dust (Psalm 104:29, 30). The story in which Elisha breathes into the boy (2 Kings 4:32-38) and the outpouring of Jesus' breath onto the disciples after the resurrection (John 20:19-31) giving them the Holy Spirit are other ways in which the Scriptures relate this truth. *Ruah* is what is divine within human beings and is that which does not go back to the dust when we die. Instead, this spirit is what passes over the line of death and returns to be with God.

Humans know only their lives in the here and now and must relate what they see and know about their world to what is revealed to them about God's world. I suggest that if we hold to the text of Scripture that says God is faithful and not arbitrary (I John 3:2), then it follows that what we see now is a foretaste of what is to come.

If the *ruah* that is within us experienced a bodily life in this world, a faithful God who could enact a resurrection is certainly capable of giving life to that human spirit after the body's death. And this is true no matter how much time we have lived before our death. I want to suggest that God does not take a child through death "early"; instead, the child grew to be all she or he was capable of being. We are each God's children in different ways. One of those ways is that we experience death at different ages. Not all of us are called to be ninety-two years old when we die. I believe it is a mistake to say that "she died too soon" or that "he died too early." I believe it is a mistake to say such things because to say them implies a judgment being made—a judgment humans ought not make. It is another way of saying "She deserved more" or "God gave me less." Such statements reflect our values and do not permit each of us to be totally unique.

God's faithfulness means that as Christ fulfilled God's will, so do we all, irrespective of our age at the time of death. The gospel according to John is replete with the phrase "When the time was fulfilled . . ." something was enacted. When time is full, something happens. There are two words for time in the Bible, one of which is *kairos*, meaning "God's time." Words which sound alike in Greek are related to one another. Another word related to *kairos* by sound is the word *cheir*, meaning "hand" (and from which the word "surgery" comes). It is a word of action as much as anatomy. When time is fulfilled, something happens. Time and death go together. At our death, our time has been fulfilled.

Adults who are parents of patients have said various versions of, "It would be different if he was in his eighties; he would have lived his whole life. Why should he have to go through this now?" Death at any age, whether elderly or juvenile, may bring with it some indignities, as anyone who has visited a nursing home can attest. I find it impossible to believe that a lengthy life justifies, or makes acceptable, some of the ways in which our elderly people die. If God does not will suffering for children, and if God is faithful, then suffering at any age should be equally abhorrent.

Some children have had a limitation (whether a physical impairment, injury, or disease), and, *in spite of that limitation,* have grown to be all they were capable of being *in this world.* Because God wills healing (wholeness), these children are brought, through the process of death, completely into God's presence. Only there are we truly made whole. The vast majority of people do not have such severe physical limitations and will not be brought into God's presence until late in their lives. The Prayers of the People in the Episcopal communion rites seek to give expression to this in the petition "We commend to your mercy all who have died, that your will for them may be fulfilled . . ." (*Book of Common Prayer,* 1979, p. 389).

Having been created out of the dust of the cosmos, at the time of death the body returns to that dust, and the *ruah* passes over from this life into an eternal life. I prefer the term Intermediate State to describe this because it lacks the emotional connotations of such words as purgatory and limbo. It also avoids words like heaven and hell, which do not exist until the Last Day. I find the New Testament to be of two minds about what happens immediately after death. Paul, as well as Mark and Matthew, describes the dead as waiting in some way for the Last Day (2 Cor 15; 1 Thes 4:13; Mk 13:26, 27 and Mt 24:30-31). Quite a different idea is put forth by Luke, who describes the dead as enjoying immediate bliss upon death (Lk 16:19-31 and 24:43). Such a contradiction posed no problem for the early church until it became clear that the immediate return of the Christ was not forthcoming. In the Anglican tradition, both of these strands of thought are considered to be within the bounds of doctrine.

The burial rite in the Episcopal tradition includes a prayer that the deceased "may go from strength to strength in the life of perfect service in your kingdom" (*Book of Common Prayer*, 1979). This is to say that the Intermediate State is not a period of dormancy, but a living and dynamic state of growth and change. It is a time of being conformed completely to God's will. This is the classical meaning of "purgation" as cleansing; it is a time during which all that is not godly about us is stripped away. It is in this state that we grow to be more God-like until the great Last Day, on which all of the faithful are clothed by God in their resurrection bodies.

This is how I have begun to think through these issues for myself. I strongly encourage anyone who works with children and teenagers to begin to reflect on these questions as well. This is not to make everyone a theologian, but because children and youth will ask questions. As a guide to begin thinking, consider how you might respond to the following questions, which were developed by a seventh-grade class in a Roman Catholic school:

- Is there such a thing as reincarnation where you could come back as someone else or live your life through someone else after dying?
- Why do people have to die?
- Where do people go when they die?
- Are you afraid of dying, and is the fear of death normal for teens to have?
- What happens after you die?
- How do we know the Bible is true?
- What is the purpose of living if we are just going to die?
- When you die, do you go to heaven, hell, or purgatory right away?
- Why can we not live forever?
- I have been told hell is a place of suffering. Is it universal suffering, an individual suffering, or just a place without being united to God?
- What happens to children if they die before they are baptized?
- Should I do everything I want now because I could die at any moment?
- How can we prepare ourselves for death?

- How can one cope with the loss of a close friend who has committed suicide—especially if this friend said he or she had thought about it?
- How can you help a teen cope with the loss of a parent?
- What if there is no God?
- Am I going to be an angel after I die?
- Are there animals in heaven?
- Can I get married when I am in heaven?

Chapter 7

Using Prayer and Rituals
with Children

Children live in a very symbolic world where all kinds of things are possible. Rituals often have great meaning to them, and my experience is that children often get more out of symbolic words and actions than adults do. It can also be true that children get more out of such rituals than *their pastoral caregivers do.* Some pastoral caregivers are reluctant to suggest any sacrament or ritual simply because it is not a valued piece of their own experience. However, a pastoral conversation with a child or youth is an opportunity to reach into and use the riches of the child's religious tradition to celebrate God's presence and love and, when necessary, to remind the youth of God's standards, mercy, and forgiveness.

Some would argue that with the rise of television's influence on children, such actions and words have little meaning left for children. I argue otherwise. The meaning of such actions may be less than in prior decades, but it is by no means gone. Many of the media characters are presented in symbolic ways, often through how they are dressed. The fear of the dark, which toddlers experience, reflects their ability to intuit that there is something outside of, and larger than, themselves. Children who are members of a worshiping community sense a rhythm through regular attendance and the passage of religious holidays. This repetition builds a sense of identity in them: "this is part of who I am." On the surface, simple attendance is a sign of belief; at a deeper level of meaning, it is also symbolic of the child's identity, relationship with God and others, and one's search for meaning and understanding.

As I will use them in this chapter, symbols are those words or actions which point to a deeper meaning or belief. Rituals or rites are spoken events in which symbolic events take place. Strictly speaking, the rite is the words themselves, which may take place in the context of a ceremony. Rituals are often associated with repetition, but this need not be so. For example, Jewish and Christian children who undergo rites of circumcision or baptism undergo them once in a lifetime. Some rituals may only have meaning for the one time they are used. Rituals such as anointing a child with oil, while laying on hands for healing prayers, may have meaning no matter how many times they are performed. Rituals are a form of speaking important truths to one another. In a religious context, the fundamental truth they normally seek to convey is of God and God's promises to humanity. Rituals are often accompanied by symbolic actions and objects. In religious communities, rituals typically occur at milestone events in lives, primarily birth, marriage, and death. Any rite of passage may be observed with a ritual so long as it conveys meaning to the child. For instance, a school-age child may well want to celebrate the new freedom of movement after a cast is removed from an arm or a leg. A family may want to celebrate the adoption of children in some way; a teenager may want to celebrate having his or her own room for the first time.

Many faith traditions have developed rituals only for a very few, common instances such as ritual circumcision, baptism, marriage, and burial. Children experience many significant life events other than these common ones. I suggest that if no ritual exists for an event in the life of a child you are pastorally related to, that you not allow this to be an excuse to let the moment pass unobserved. In these cases, exercise your creativity and develop what is needed. The origin of such a ritual may be a comment heard during an informal conversation in which a child or youth mentions an upcoming significant event. The pastoral person can affirm the child's feeling and offer to observe that occasion with the child so that God can join in the celebration. For many children, the notion that God takes delight in the simple events of their lives will come as a surprise. This is an opportunity to teach people that what we give thanks for, we make sacred. So inviting God into the events of their lives is a natural event.

Except for rituals of birth, marriage, and death, the pastoral person has a wide range of places in which to celebrate the ritual.

Natural options would include the child's home or within the congregation at some time other than during the public worship services. Good rituals are succinct. Write the words that convey what you believe God celebrates or mourns in this event in the form of a prayer. You may add a simple lesson from a holy book that applies. Rituals normally use something from the natural world to serve as a reminder of God's presence and promise. Water may be appropriate for sprinkling or blessing; wine, if eating or drinking is to be symbolized; and olive oil is also used to mark people who are special, or in special need of God's healing and care. These are very traditional items. You may consider using balloons or other items at funerals. If both the child and the parents are to be involved, it may be appropriate for them to give a symbolic gift to one another. Although rituals do not normally take a long time to celebrate, they do require some creativity and forethought. Creativity is an expression of God's Spirit within us. Celebrating rites with children are times to allow the Spirit to work in new ways:

> Nellie is an ordained Protestant pastor in a large, downtown congregation. In relating a visit with Omar, a seven-year-old boy hospitalized after a simple surgery, she confessed that at the end of the visit she did not know what to do. "I felt like I should say a prayer, but I did not know what words to use—simple words, as if I were Omar talking to God, or my own words, which Omar might not get as much out of. So I ended up just patting him on the head and saying, 'God bless you.'"

Nellie's experience brings up a number of issues. Prayer and ritual contribute to making a pastoral visit unique among all of the other visitors that a child will have. How to handle them, though, raises some questions. It is a good idea to adjust the language of any ritual so that it is meaningful to the participants. In the case of children, this means adjusting what you say to their level. If the children are school-age, watch the number of multisyllable words, and seek to use simple sentences rather than complex or compound ones. Using the rule that prayer is our talking to God, then perhaps Nellie's most appropriate prayer would have talked to God in the same way she hopefully spoke with Omar. If our conversation with children is adjusted to be close to their level, then our conversation with God most closely expresses what is in a child's heart when we speak to God on that same level. The same principle holds true if a pastoral caregiver is writing a ritual to use at a later time. If finding the right kind of words for developing a prayer or ritual is difficult, one might find and read several religious books written for children about the same age as you are working with to see how they address and talk about God.

Experiment and suggest to the children in your care that you join with them in celebrating the many little turning points in their lives. The remainder of this chapter is devoted to some of the more commonly encountered situations. This is not to limit your creativity in any way.

BAPTISM OF CHILDREN

> Pastor Peter received a telephone call in his office from a frantic new member whose newborn appeared to need cardiac surgery within the next two days. The new father asked the pastor to come to the hospital and baptize the child before the surgery.

"Would you baptize our child?" is not an uncommon request for a minister to be confronted with when an infant is suddenly hospitalized or is likely to have surgery. Baptism is understood to be a rite by which a person enters the community of believers and receives full membership into the Christian community. The communal nature of the rite has been increasingly emphasized. Baptisms that take place at other times and in other places than the regular worship life of the congregation, such as baptisms in hospitals, are presumed to be emergent situations with at least a possible, if not probable, chance that the person will die soon.

My experience in talking with teenagers and parents of ill infants is that fear is the greatest underlying source of motivation in requesting the rite. It is important that pastoral care not only help the child experience God but also address the underlying emotion that is moving the child to reach out to God at this time. Without having that discussion, ordained clergy reduce themselves to being mere "technicians of the sacraments" who perform their liturgical office and depart with few extra words spoken. It may even be that the rite is not what people want. Sometimes, though, baptism is a name they know to ask for when they are feeling scared or desperate and want *something* done:

> Quinten was sixteen years old and hospitalized for leukemia after a relapse from his remission. He was increasingly uncomfortable and knew that he would not live much longer. Late one night he asked his nurse to page the chaplain; upon the chaplain's arrival, Quinten asked to be baptized. The chaplain knew some of Quinten's history and knew that while Quinten believed in God, he did not believe in Christ, and neither he nor his parents had been members of any congregation in many years.

Quinten's story is typical in that fear was the motivation to make this request. When faced with a request like his, my response is, "Well, we can certainly talk about that. You seem pretty anxious. I am wondering if you can tell me what it is that you are most afraid of right now?" The responses may seem rather obvious; common ones are the fear of death (or of dying) and the fear of being imminently judged by God. When the request is put forward by the parent of an infant or newborn, the fear is often the fear that the child may not be with God in heaven. Sometimes this conversation provides an opportunity for persons (either teenage patients or parents of a young child) to unburden themselves from a guilt or sin they have been carrying for a long time.

Helping people articulate the fears provides the pastoral caregiver with an opportunity to provide some simple education about the church's beliefs and practices. It might also be an opportunity to read some brief passages of Scripture that talk about how God might receive people when they die, whether that is today or in eighty years. Which passages the pastoral visitor chooses to select and how one explains the church's beliefs will differ with every pastoral caregiver.

Since the circumstances surrounding a baptism are assumed to be special, the pastoral caregiver might carry that out in some unique ways. Hospital rites of all kinds tend to be simple in nature because they often take place in an emergent situation. It is important to remember, though, that this is the only baptism that this child will experience, and the pastoral caregiver should work to make it as meaningful as possible. I believe in using a number of concrete items when I perform a baptism, which I then give to the child (or the parents if the child is an infant). The first of these is a large collection of shells, which someone who vacationed at a beach brought back for me. In some hospitals, a nurse will be able to obtain a small plastic bottle of sterile water for the baptism; some pastoral caregivers prefer to bring their own. I always pour the water into the shell and use that to baptize the child. A women's group made simple baptismal napkins, which I then use to dry the child's head and face. These are another way in which one might involve a larger portion of the congregation into one's pastoral ministry, as these are simply made from a white cloth. Both of these items and a baptismal certificate serve as concrete reminders to the children of what they have been through.

If baptism by immersion is the custom in the patient's tradition, this can often be carried out even in a hospital setting. Immersion baptisms require some advance notice and cooperation with the hospital's health care team. They may be quite surprised at the need for immersion rather than mere sprinkling, and explaining that this is the patient's request will be helpful. One objection that may be raised is that there are central lines or other items that may not get wet. If the staff is supportive of the patient's request, though, even this objection can be overcome.

Frequently, hospitals will have a whirlpool or tub located in the physical therapy unit that is large enough to immerse a person in. If the hospital has a burn center, there will certainly be tubs large enough for this purpose. Last, hospital employee fitness centers may have a swimming pool that may be used. If baptism by immersion is desired, the pastoral caregiver may let the child or youth know that this opportunity will be looked into. The hospital chaplain, if one is available, will be aware of what resources are available and can facilitate making the arrangements. If there is no chaplain, the nurse in charge of the unit where the patient is should be the next person with whom to discuss this issue.

NAMING CEREMONIES

A naming ceremony may be appropriate in cases where baptism is to be deferred until the child is healthy enough or old enough for the rite to take place in a congregation. It may also be an option when baptism is not considered appropriate due to the patient's age, medical condition (including cases where the child has or will imminently die), or the pastoral caregiver's own discomfort over the child or family member's ability to fulfill the baptismal covenant. In such cases, a naming ceremony may be suggested as an alternative. This is not to demean it to a second-class status but as an alternative that more closely expresses one's wishes. The reason for deferring or withholding baptism should be clearly stated. Then the pastoral person can acknowledge hearing the fear, anxiety, or other emotion, and the naming ceremony may be offered as a means of bringing this child and the child's desires to God. The rite for naming a child that follows is meant to be a framework and may be suitably altered to fit the circumstances.

The pastor begins with this opening prayer:

Eternal God, you spoke your name to Moses so that we might know you and draw near to you as your children and not as strangers. You bid us call you, and abide with you. Hear us as we gather to name your servant before you this day that this child may be known to us as powerfully as *she* is known to you.

Everyone responds:

Amen.

One of the following readings or some other suitable reading may be used:

Moses said to God, "If I come to the Israelites and say to them, 'The God of your ancestors has sent me to you,' and they ask me, 'What is his name?' what shall I say to them?" God said to Moses, "I AM WHO I AM." (Exodus 3:13-14a, NRSV)

Jesus said, "I am the good shepherd. I know my own and my own know me, just as the Father knows me and I know the Father." (John 10:14-15a, NRSV)

A brief homily or reflection on God's presence in and through this child may take place. If a biblical name or one with other religious meaning is given, the pastor may give its meaning or talk about the qualities of the biblical character.

The pastor then asks the gathered family members the following:

God knows this child more deeply than we can imagine. By what name will you know this child in your hearts and lives?

When the child, if old enough to speak for himself or herself, or the family members have given the name, the pastor says the following or similar words:

N.M., we rejoice to recognize you as a child of God. Naming you opens the way for those who love you to carry your identity with them, for you to be as present with them when they call on you as you are always present to God.

Let us pray.

Everloving God, we thank you for N.M., and for sending her into this family to know and to love. Grant that their love for N.M. may be a glimpse of the love you have for each one of us.

Everyone responds:

Amen.

ANOINTING CHILDREN WITH OIL

Sacramental rites are used because they are aids to our memories. They use an element from the natural world to help us feel God's presence and to remind us of God's promises and love. Anointing those who are ill with oil and praying over them finds its scriptural warrants in the anointing of the kings of Israel as a sign of God's raising them to this office and in the letter of James (5:14), which admonishes the sick to call for the elders of the church to pray over them and anoint them with oil in the name of the Lord. As outlined in that letter, the act of anointing and praying by members of the community of faith recalls God's love for each person and God's promises of wholeness and salvation:

> Rae was a fourteen-year-old girl admitted to the hospital's psychiatric unit for anorexia. She and her family attended a Roman Catholic parish. In a conversation about the rituals of the church, she asked, "Am I sick enough to be anointed?"

This is a rite that may be offered to any child at any time; it is also a rite that may be beneficial even if it is not normally a part of the child's religious tradition. Far too often is this rite neglected, either because it is not one of the two that Jesus actually performed or because of its association with Last Rites and death. The Roman Catholic Church now refers to this rite as the Sacrament of the Sick, which emphasizes that it is for the living. This rite in the Roman Catholic Church has been associated with penitence and reconciliation; hence, there has been a reluctance on the part of many priests to anoint children who have not yet attained the age of reason.

I believe that this is a rite from which many persons can benefit. I also believe that it is a rite that requires some forethought and, many times, some explanation. This is especially true if the rite is not common in the pastoral visitor's tradition. Healing, however, is a quality to be sought on all levels: body, mind, and spirit. Prayer for healing should always be accompanied by actions that promote healing and health: heathy diet, exercise, and seeking medical and/or psychiatric care when appropriate. It is also important to distinguish between healing and cure. Sometimes cure is not possible. And some of what needs healing in our lives are the broken relationships and the hurts caused by our words and actions. Healing is much broader than cure. Although God is not a genie to be conjured up to perform the feats we desire, God does want to hear the prayers and cries that are on our hearts and lips. Prayers for cures, even miraculous ones, are not inappropriate when we realize that sometimes the only way for someone to be made whole is to be brought directly into God's presence through death.

Human life inevitably involves suffering. Life in this world is not perfect, and, therefore, we can gain something by being with God. Anointing with oil and praying for healing is part of what God's people always do: they gather to pray, to acknowledge that there is brokenness in our lives, and to ask God to heal those parts of life that are broken.

Each year on Maundy Thursday, the clergy of our diocese gather with the bishop to renew our ordination vows. During that service, olive oil that will be given to clergy to use to anoint the sick and the newly baptized is blessed. I also drop one or two spice cloves in my small bottle of oil, which gives it a wonderful aroma. When I talk to children about anointing, I explain to them that long after I have left them, they might notice this smell "sort of like oranges or something from your kitchen" hovering around you even though you cannot see it. This smell is a reminder of God's presence and God's Spirit hovering around you even though you cannot see God. God is as close to you as this smell. Many times I find that it is not only the child's face that lights up but the parents' faces as well.

One of the differences between children and adults is the sense of their own bodies. Adults tend to relate to God primarily with their intellect—or at least, they can hear themselves talk to God in their minds. And so when it comes to anointing, most adults will find it quite natural for pastoral visitors to put oil and lay their hands on patients' foreheads during prayer. Children tend to be more focused on a specific body part. If you are going to use oil to anoint a child, ask the child's permission to put the oil on the part of the body that hurts or is broken. You might phrase this with a statement such as, "I would like to put some oil where you would like God's healing to touch you. Can you show me where that might be?" Any part of the body that is normally covered by a bathing suit should not be anointed because of sexual boundary issues. In those cases, one might offer to anoint the forehead as with an adult or the back of the child's hand. The place where children want God to touch them most may not be the obvious body part either! This was brought home to me while visiting the nine-year-old boy who was hospitalized for appendicitis. It was far more important to him that God's healing be directed toward the bruise on his arm from a Little League baseball game than to the incision on his abdomen. Since that encounter, I always ask children where they would like to be anointed!

FUNERALS AND CHILDREN

There are two separate issues here: children attending funerals and funerals of children. Each of these will be considered individually.

Children Attending Funerals

> Samantha's father had just died in the nursing home where he had lived for several years. Most of the family had gathered to be with him including her two children, ages six and nine. Samantha's pastor was also present and raised the issue of planning the funeral. Samantha looked troubled and said, "I guess we could do it Wednesday morning while the kids are in school. Or do you think they should be there?"

This is a question that many clergy hear. Children who are old enough to love, and that certainly includes toddlers, are old enough to grieve and to express their feelings. Yet many times I have heard family members say, "Oh, they are too young to understand!" Young children may lack the vocabulary to talk about their feelings or death, but their behaviors indicate that they understand that a significant change has taken place. A change in sleep habits, regressive behaviors, and explosive emotions are all possible ways in which younger children will show their grief. Pastoral caregivers might prepare families to experience this and suggest that hugging and holding the children are ways to support them while they mourn. Attending the funeral is as much an opportunity for them to mourn as it is for adults. One of the ways in which children learn is through modeling adult behaviors. They need to learn that the feelings their parents may be showing are normal and acceptable. Perhaps they may need to learn that such feelings are not their fault; they are not responsible for their parents' feelings. If children see adults openly displaying their feelings, they learn that this is an acceptable coping skill to have and use. If children learn good grieving at a young age, they will have these skills for the rest of their lives and experience fewer complications in mourning in the future.

Having children who are between the ages of four and thirteen present does call for some pastoral work before the funeral. I am indebted to the Reverend Dr. Edward Kryder for the following metaphors to explain burials to children. A good response to Samantha's question in the previous vignette might run along the lines of, "I really think it is important for your children to be present. I would like to meet with them and talk with them before the service begins. I want to talk with them about what they will see and hear during the service for their grandfather. I wonder if you might be able to come about a half hour early?"

My primary goal during this meeting is to dispel any notions that we are burying the *person* rather than the body. For this meeting, I have sat on the floor, either at the foot of the altar steps or in the funeral home in the room in which the funeral will take place, with the children of the family seated around me. This does not have to be a private meeting with the children, and sometimes the adults who are present will be able to hear the explanations and metaphors. They may remember and use them later when the children have questions about the service or the person who died.

I bring the robes I will wear during the service to this gathering, although I do not put them on until later. After the initial introductions, I ask them what they expect to happen. One child will usually say, "We are going to put grandfather (or whomever) in the ground!" This is the opening I look for because it gives me the opportunity to say, "I want to be very clear with you. There is one thing we are *not* going to do today, and that is to put your grandfather into the ground." At this point I hold up the robe and stole that I brought and relate that these are very important clothes to me. I have had a lot of good times in them. I have celebrated many services for many people while I was wearing them, and I remember those persons when I put these clothes on. One day, though, they will wear out and become so frayed and ragged that I will not be able to use them anymore. These clothes are so precious that when that day comes, I will not let my wife just throw them into the rag box. I will treat them and get rid of them in a special way. This service we are about to have is not about burying a person. This person's body has worn out because it was well-used for a long time. Since this person was very special, we treat his or her body in a special way and that is by putting it into a special container called a casket and putting that casket into the ground.

If the person who died has been cremated, one can alter the end of the explanation to include the idea that burning a body turns it into ashes, which are put in a special container and then put in a special place. I have found that it is better to use words such as container rather than box when talking about a casket. Children have very clear ideas about what a box is from having played in them and may well get the wrong idea. Sufficient time should be given for the children to ask any questions they might have.

Funeral of a Child

This is one of the pastoral events about which more clergy have expressed unease (and even fear) about having to preside over. Although by this point I do not believe the child is in further need of our assistance, a meaningful funeral is still part of providing sound pastoral care to the child, because we care about him or her. For those traditions that include prayers to, or on behalf of, the dead, the words of the burial service are believed to have power and meaning as well.

I strongly suggest that pastoral caregivers consider a back-to-front order for the funeral of infants and children. In this case, the service begins at the graveside (or wherever the ashes are being committed). Generally this takes place with immediate family and perhaps a few close friends present. Ideally, the grave would be closed immediately upon conclusion of the graveside service while the family is present. The funeral service would follow, ideally in the congregation, and this would be followed by a reception or simple luncheon put on by a group in the congregation. This luncheon provides a place for people to gather, to tell stories, and to celebrate the child's life.

The advantage of doing the service in this order is that it begins with the finality of burying the body, moves to a funeral service that is a celebration of the child's life, and ends with a more informal celebration and sharing of memories. Although the family will certainly be openly grieving during this time, this order avoids having them sit through the funeral service staring at the casket thinking about what must come next. Parents have told me that the thought of the actual committal and burial was so strong that they did not hear the funeral service itself and were not always aware of who was present to support them. Clearly, arranging the order to begin with the graveside will require significant more preparation by the pastoral caregiver. It is untraditional enough that it requires a high level of trust of the pastoral caregiver by the family. Closing the grave immediately is no longer the norm in some cemeteries, and morticians and cemetery superintendents may be reluctant to do things in this way unless the clergyperson can speak to the reasons why this is proposed. The reluctance on the part of morticians and cemetery administrators to assist with such arrangements may stem from their own fears about "what might happen" to the family. The pastoral caregiver can work with such people to help them understand the importance of doing a funeral in this way, emphasizing that care of the family is the pastoral caregiver's responsibility.

Some other options that the priest might want to offer for families' consideration include a launching of balloons. This might take place outside the congregation after the funeral or from the graveside itself. It is yet another way to symbolize the child's new union with God, and it is a way to involve other children who attend the service. Inclusion and participation allow them to have a ritual way to display and deal with their emotions. Planting a tree in the child's memory is also a possibility. This could be done at any time and even take place months or years after the death. A pastoral person might create a simple rite of prayers remembering the child and the digging of a hole and planting and watering the new tree. If siblings of the child who died are present, the pastoral caregiver might meet with them and plan the service with their help. Who wants to read a Bible story? What do you want to pray about? Who wants to bring water to the tree? And so on. This can become a genuine family service.

The task of preaching at the funeral of a child is daunting to many of us who have been called upon to do so. The pressures are enormous: it is a highly emotional event; the preacher feels a strong need to make sense of a tragedy; noncongregational members are present whom the preacher would also like to reach with the text; and the preacher's own ability to make sense of the events may cause pressure. All of these combine to make this a formidable task. A question I am frequently asked by clergy is, "What do I say?" The first pointer is to *use the child's name.* Parents *need* to hear their child's name spoken aloud because that child was real. Many of the parents' friends and family will avoid using the child's name due to the pain of remembering it: this is an opportunity for the pastoral caregiver to model a healing behavior. The second pointer is to give the parents a copy of whatever written text or note cards the preacher uses. Parents have reported to me that they read and reread the funeral sermons for strength for weeks after the service. The service will certainly be a time of high emotion for them, and they simply will not hear and absorb every word the preacher says. Having a written copy of it allows them to go back and pick up what they missed and to continue to ponder the words. The following is a model for sermons at the funeral for a child:

> I met N two years ago, shortly after he was diagnosed with cancer at the hospital. We soon discovered a common interest in baseball and talked about our favorite teams. He had a real passion for the local team. As time went on, we talked of other things, about how he looked forward to turning sixteen and that it meant he would soon be able to drive and where he would go and who he would take along. Eventually our conversations turned to N's ideas and images of God and the afterlife and whether there were cars he could drive in heaven and ball teams to cheer on.
>
> As our time together increased, I quickly became attached to N, and I have found myself wanting to cling, to hold on to him. You can imagine a child in the womb wanting to stay put. After all, it is a warm and safe and known place. And then comes this strange experience called birth. Being born can be wrenching for the child, being suddenly pushed out into a place that is very different and cold and bright. In that newness, however, there is something beautiful and better—life—on the other side.

Later in N's life, he was baptized. The grace that is poured out in baptism does not come from anything any one of us did; instead, its grace is something that God does. The water that was poured out was not "magic dust." Baptism did recognize N as belonging to God and meant that his spirit was the Spirit of God within him. One of the things we can be certain about is that we do not escape sadness or suffering by being baptized, or by being Christian. Our faith is not an insurance policy that protects us from illness or pain.

N's baptism means that as part of God's fellowship that relationship of love continues after death. It was dying that brought N before the throne of God. Dying, in some ways, is like being born. N moved from a place that was warm and safe and known to someplace new—being with God.

Like the child in the womb, we may want to cling, to hold on to N. We do not know what came next for him, but we can trust in God that there is something beautiful and better—eternal life—on the other side. One of the things we can be certain about is that God is not finished with N yet. God promised that all who love God share God's nature and will never die eternally. N will continue to grow in knowledge and understanding and love. The afterlife is life, and one in which we carry on growing and learning.

If you have ever looked at the back of a tapestry, you know that it is a mess. There are knots and loose ends and threads running every which way. You can only get a glimpse of the beauty and pattern and order that is on the other side. Our earthly life is very much like being on the back of a tapestry. There are lots of knots and unfinished business and unanswered questions. Only N, on the other side, can fully see and appreciate the pattern and beauty and order that is there.

Death is a mystery for us still. And that is hard. It makes our loss real, and strong, and painful. Perhaps it is a blessing that we do not know all that there is. Perhaps it is a good thing that we cannot see the afterlife yet, because so much of what we can see in this life is not easy to look at. If we could picture being with God, it might look a little too much like earth, and heaven is not something we can create; it is something God has created. And it is therefore more wonderful than we can imagine or dream of.

Rather than picture something that looks too much like earth, we have instead the promise of God, made real in baptism, of eternal life with God. And we have the image of Jesus embracing little children and drawing them to himself. Jesus welcomed children on earth. I have no doubt that he welcomed N into his heavenly life and is with him right now.

Reverse side imagery, such as the previous tapestry example, is one way of expressing the feelings of not understanding the tragedy. Another possibility is the back of a mirror, which is silvered or dusted; from that side, one can only see outlines or shapes on the other side. Or the example of hoarfrost appearing on windows in the winter, which makes delicate and intricate patterns and which disappears with the rising of the sun. A young adult with ALS (Lou Gehrig's disease) once told me that she imagined herself as a stone sculpture that was a work still in progress. As the piece of sculpture, she herself could not see where the blows were originating from, she could only feel them when they struck (and sometimes see them coming). What she could not see was the beauty that was emerging from the work; that was not her perspective. At some point she would be able to stand on the other side, and from that perspective she fully expected to be able to see the completed work in the same context that God saw her. It is a reverse side image of a different sort, and one that emphasizes the amount of trust in the sculptor, that patients with chronic and terminal illnesses can call upon to support them through these illnesses.

Caring for Children After Any Death

There is often a sense among adults that something needs to be done for children after a death. Sometimes this manifests in rushes to overprotect them from emotional pain, and sometimes it is merely the projection of the adults' own sense of helplessness onto the most obviously weak and vulnerable family members. It may be that the best care the pastoral person can provide for the children is to protect them from either of these extremes, and create an environment where kids are allowed to be kids.

At some point shortly after a death, a brief overview of grief can be shared with the child's parents. Contemporary North American culture is one that denies and hides death from view. Many adults have consequently never mourned someone when they were children and are unable to recognize the very real but very different ways in which children mourn and grieve. The basic sketch to give to parents includes mention of the fact that children mourn differently. They mourn in small doses and they mourn for a longer period of time. Adults frequently are unaware of this dynamic and mistake a child's grief for lack of feelings, or awareness, or even call it denial. In doing so they miss the opportunity to talk with their children about death and about the person who has died.

The primary difference in how children grieve is the duration. As adults, we tend to do most of our crying during the period immediately after a death, and as time goes on, it diminishes quickly. Children, by contrast, mourn in doses, which is to say they mourn for a *short* period (literally as short as three to five minutes). Afterward, they may show no outward signs of grief for a period of time that might be several hours to days. And unlike adults, who have largely done most of their open mourning during the first weeks after the death, a child's mourning will frequently continue in these short doses for a year or more. A child might mourn very obviously through tears, but it may also come out in play. Crashing toy cars together and then forming a funeral procession; stuffed animals consoling each other; or burying objects in a sandbox or in the ground are all ways in which young children might reenact all or part of a death or funeral. A pastoral caregiver might prepare a family to see this or inquire whether they have seen it, and assure them this is normal and expected. Even when the death is of an adult and no children are present, if the pastoral caregiver is aware of children or grandchildren in the family constellation, it would be a pastoral act to draw their attention to the different ways children grieve.

If the adults are mourning in healthy ways, chances are very good that the children will mourn in healthy ways as well, and move on with their lives. Understanding what is unique to children and permission for children to have their different ways of being will certainly aid in this process.

Annotated Bibliography

This book is a device to help pastoral caregivers on their way toward delivering meaningful pastoral care without being overcome by their anxiety and without projecting it onto the children. In addition to the specific references I have cited in my text, I have included in this bibliography many books that I have found most influential in my formation as a pastoral person. Not all of them are explicitly religious; not all of them are directly about pastoral care. Although all pastoral caregivers will develop their own favorite resources, this may serve as a list of recommended topics and titles to pursue in the future.

NARRATIVES ABOUT ILLNESS

Bombeck, Erma (1989). *I Want to Grow Hair, I Want to Grow Up, I Want to Go to Boise.* New York: Harper and Row.

The author lets children who are cancer survivors tell their stories. It is all here—the playfulness, the resilience, and the fears. Having read this book, pastoral caregivers are less likely to project their values and beliefs onto the patients and families. It is also a good catalyst for learning how to invite children to tell their stories. There are also a number of drawings done by the children; for pastoral caregivers unfamiliar with drawing and talking, these can serve as examples of what might be encountered. This book provides a glimpse into the world of children coping with an illness that frightens most adults.

Dubuque, Susan E. (1996). *A Parent's Survival Guide to Childhood Depression.* King of Prussia, PA: The Center for Applied Psychology.

This wonderful book uses the images of "turtles" and "dragons" to describe how many girls and boys display their depression. Reading this book will help pastoral caregivers empathize with what parents whose children have depression experience when they are being diagnosed and learning to live with this illness. It is also an excellent book to recommend to parents; it may help them feel less isolated and may teach them about treatment options, coping with their own stress, and how to help their child.

Spufford, Margaret (1996). *Celebration: A Story of Joy and Suffering.* Cambridge, MA: Cowley Publications.

This is a first-person account of a mother and daughter who have chronic, debilitating conditions, and the daughter's was terminal. This is the story of a woman who refused to accept the lame explanations for suffering and evil that are too easily pandered by well-meaning but ultimately meaningless clergy and physicians. In the process of telling their two stories, the author articulates the agony and the questions and begins to develop her own answers.

Styron, William (1990). *Darkness Visible.* New York: Random House.

Subtitled "A Memoir of Madness," this is a first-person account by a Pulitzer Prize-winning author of his experiences of being clinically depressed and suicidal. He vividly describes his descent into the throes of depression, his hospitalization, and recovery. Reading this book is perhaps the nearest a pastoral caregiver can get to understanding mental illness without actually living through it.

PRAYER AND RITUALS WITH CHILDREN

(1979). *The Book of Common Prayer.* New York: Seabury Press.

This is the book of rites and ceremonies of the Episcopal Church. Several of the rites pertain directly to children, including the rite for Thanksgiving for the Birth or Adoption of a Child. There are also specific prayers for use when children are ill and suggestions for readings and planning the funeral of a child.

Brooke, Avery (1996). *Healing in the Landscape of Prayer.* Cambridge, MA: Cowley Publications.

A solid introductory book for persons interested in beginning a healing ministry within a church. The author covers the history of healing within the church and then looks at a variety of prayer experiences. She outlines how a healing ministry can be developed and nurtured in a congregation based on the variety of prayer experiences and how one's inner healing is a part of this process. A comparison between New Age healing and Christian healing is drawn. The bibliography on healing is excellent.

Ward, Hannah and Jennifer Wild (1995). *Human Rites.* London: Mowbray.

The compilers have collected or written rites, prayers, and hymns for a wide variety of life events—often events that are not observed by mainline churches but that are significant in the lives of persons. Included are naming ceremonies, funeral liturgies for cases of miscarriage, stillborn children and infant death, as well as baptism, coming-of-age ceremonies, and many others. A helpful resource from which to borrow language for one's own prayers even if the rites are not used as written.

CHILDREN AND GOD

Capps, Donald J. (1995). *The Child's Song.* Louisville, KY: Westminster John Knox Press.

Subtitled "The Religious Abuse of Children," the author outlines how the Bible and religious authority figures have abused children, especially emotionally, in the past. It is also a book about healing—healing the child within the pastoral caregiver whose own growth toward God may have been stunted—and about how to live as a pastor so that the children we care for are not hurt by our ministries.

Coles, Robert (1990). *The Spiritual Life of Children.* Boston, MA: Houghton Mifflin.

There are some books that, if you are going to work in the field, you have to read. This is one of those books. For anyone interested in doing pastoral care with children, this book is an important foundation. Based upon his extensive conversations with children of various religious traditions, the author describes what children believe and how their beliefs are shaped. Although he does not use the language of seeing children as a gift, he nevertheless models a way of listening to children's voices and valuing what they say. The author clearly demonstrates that children indeed have rich spiritual lives, although they do not use the same vocabulary as adults to describe them.

Erikson, Erik H. (1963). *Childhood and Society,* Second Edition. New York: W.W. Norton and Company.

Erikson's neo-Freudian work on how children develop includes the idea that society molds and shapes a child's development. Erikson conceives of a child's development as successfully negotiating a series of crises, beginning with the ability to trust others (or not). This work remains a classic in child development.

Fowler, James W. (1981). *Stages of Faith.* San Francisco: Harper and Row.

Fowler's book is based upon extensive research conversations with people about what gives meaning to their lives. In this book, faith is equated with meaning and a person's values. It is not necessarily a religious word. He describes six stages of faith. It is tempting, but misleading, to conceive of them as discrete steps. It may be better to talk about a person demonstrating the behavior of a particular stage, as opposed to that person being in a particular stage. This is an excellent book that begins to truly blend meaning with contemporary psychology.

Fuhrmann, Barbara Schneider (1986). *Adolescence, Adolescents.* Boston, MA: Little, Brown, and Company.

If one were to own only one book that covered developmental ideas and neatly outlined the issues that confront adolescents, this would be it. The introductions to the work of Piaget, Erikson, Kohlberg and others are readable. The chapters on religious development and moral education are excellent. Together, these chapters help one understand how to shape questions and hear the concerns and the underlying reasons that adolescents face. One section covers psychiatric disorders, substance abuse issues, and gangs.

Oppenheimer, Helen (1995). *Helping Children Find God.* Harrisburg, PA: Morehouse Publishing.

Subtitled "A Book for Parents, Teachers, and Clergy," this book presents a way to encourage children's natural curiosity in ways that lead them to God. She demonstrates how God can be found in many places, including nature, other people, churches, and in the Bible. Conversations and reflection lead children to experiencing and building relationships with God. An excellent reference book for anyone who works with children and is interested in being with them as they build relationships with God. This would also make a fine gift for parents when a child is baptized or confirmed.

DEATH AND DYING

Heegaard, Marge (1988). *When Someone Very Special Dies.* Minneapolis, MN: Woodland Press.

This is a coloring book for children, ages six through twelve, to work their way through the many feelings they have after someone they love dies. The only additional material required is a simple box of crayons. This would make an ideal medium for a pastoral caregiver to "drop by" and visit with, inviting the child to color and talk as they work. As children choose what to color and how, the pastoral caregiver can help them give voice to what they are feeling. Not an explicitly religious book, it still provides an excellent starting point for conversations about death, God, and an afterlife. A facilitator's guide is available.

Kübler-Ross, Elisabeth (1969). *On Death and Dying.* New York: Collier Books.

One of the first works published about what the dying have to say about their experience. Based upon interviews with dying patients, the author went on to outline "stages" of the dying process. Since the publication of this book, the attitudes of many caregivers have changed so that persons are understood to be capable of being in more than one stage at a time, and that moving out of the sequence described by the author is a normal tendency. Nonetheless, this book remains influential and deserves to remain so for the model it adopts of listening to persons describe and give meaning to their experience.

Mitchell, Joni (1969). "Woodstock."

This song proclaims a truth about our origins. Precisely because it is not in the Scriptures, this song may be used with teens to begin a discussion about creation and about death and dying. Listening to this song can be an effective introduction to these subjects. Even without a background in astronomy, pastoral caregivers can begin by asking what teens think about being equal with others and about being created from dust.

Nouwen, Henri (1982). *A Letter of Consolation.* San Francisco, CA: Harper and Row.

A classic book expressing very clearly the feelings of a man grieving his mother's death. This slender book provides excellent material for reflecting on what one believes about death and God.

Oppenheimer, Helen (1988). *The Hope of Heaven.* Cambridge, MA: Cowley Publications.

The variety of concepts about what the afterlife will be like abound. Not all of the them are scripturally sound, however. This volume, written by an Anglican lay theologian, presents a very biblically based view of what heaven is (and is not). She addresses the flaws inherent in many contemporary views. Each chapter ends with short passages from literature and Scripture for further reflection. In addition to being very helpful for wrestling with one's ideas about death and the afterlife, this book would also make an excellent text for an adult or teenage discussion class.

PASTORAL CARE

Association of Professional Chaplains. *Code of Ethics.* Schaumberg, IL: Association of Professional Chaplains.

This Code of Ethics was developed for pastoral caregivers in a specialized setting, yct the principles it articulates for confidentiality apply to anyone who engages in pastoral care.

Bolton, Robert (1979). *People Skills.* New York: Touchstone Books.

Everyone thinks they have good people skills; the reality is that most people's could be improved. This book teaches communication skills that help the pastor develop "the third ear" for listening carefully to what others are saying. The section on attending and reflecting skills is excellent. Quality pastoral care is built in part on clear, open, healthy communication. The author discusses open-ended questions and provides examples that demonstrate how these skills are useful in pastoral conversations.

Clebsch, William A. and Charles R. Jaekle (1964). *Pastoral Care in Historical Perspective.* Englewood Cliffs, NJ: Prentice-Hall.

A book primarily interesting to the historian rather than the practitioner, this book shows how pastoral care has been understood and offered over centuries in the Christian churches. I make reference to it primarily for the definition of pastoral care that is developed in it.

Detwiler-Zapp, Diane and William Caveness Dixon (1982). *Lay Caregiving.* Philadelphia, PA: Fortress Press.

This short book is a practical guidebook for those interested in developing a group of lay persons for pastoral caregiving. Sections are devoted to the theological foundation for lay caregiving, the recruitment of suitable persons, and their ongoing needs for support and training. Although it does not specifically address using teenagers as caregivers, the material presented would clearly lend itself to use with youth.

Fowler, James W. (1987). *Faith Development and Pastoral Care*. Philadelphia, PA: Fortress Press.

Part of a series on theology and pastoral care, this book begins with a definition of pastoral care, which I have reflected upon in my text. The definition is broad and centered very strongly in the context of one's worshiping community. Fowler is concerned not only with children but with the provision of pastoral care throughout the lifespan. It is not necessary to have read *Stages of Faith* before this book; for most practitioners, the discussion of each stage here will be sufficient.

Fulton, Ruth Ann B. and Carol Murphy Moore (1995). Spiritual care of the school-age child with a chronic condition. *Journal of Pediatric Nursing*, 10(4) (August), pp. 224-231.

This article, written by and for nurses, presents a definition of chronic condition to which I refer in my text. There are also short but helpful sections in this article about the use of play and about appropriate self-disclosure.

Gilbert, Binford W. (1998). *The Pastoral Care of Depression*. Binghamton, NY: The Haworth Pastoral Press.

The author wrote this book to stress teaching pastoral caregivers about depression. A clear outline of depression is presented, and how to think through alternatives before approaching people to suggest they seek help. The chapter on cognitive therapy provides a basic foundation; having this knowledge would put the pastoral caregiver in a better position to support the care and treatment that an adolescent in the congregation is receiving. Although no explicit mention of teenagers and children is made, this book still serves as a solid, single-volume introduction to providing pastoral care for people who have depression.

Holst, Lawrence E., Ed. (1996). *Hospital Ministry*. New York: Crossroad Publishing Company.

The author presents a definition of pastoral care to which I make reference in my text. This book is intended primarily to examine the contemporary role of chaplains in hospitals. The chapter (written by a different author) about pediatric care is also useful to caregivers who are not chaplains.

> Niklas, Gerald R. (1981). *The Making of a Pastoral Person.* New York: Alba House.

This is a wonderful one-volume presentation of how someone develops into being someone's pastor. The author looks at feelings, authority, anger, sexuality, and group process as elements that pastors must confront if their ministries are to move beyond the superficial. There is an excellent treatment of Erikson's stages of development from a theological perspective that is concrete, readable, and helpful in understanding how to talk with children about God. The concluding chapter is on the spirituality of the pastor.

> Nouwen, Henri (1972). *The Wounded Healer.* Garden City, NJ: Doubleday.

Probably the best-known work by this prolific author, and the book that began to help clergy deal with their own identities as caregivers based upon their own brokenness. Rather than seek to cover up problems, the author argues that is the caregivers' own problems that allow for empathy to be experienced and expressed. In developing his point, the author deals with the causes of suffering and brokenness and deals with issues of theodicy in a simple and biblically grounded way.

> Pruyser, Paul W. (1976). *The Minister As Diagnostician.* Philadelphia, PA: Westminster Press.

This classic book was developed by a clinical psychologist working with psychiatric patients who argues that pastoral caregivers can evaluate and diagnose problems in religious or spiritual language. The chapter on forging a partnership with other health professionals is very good. The chapter on pastoral diagnosis provides an array of questions to set the context for a person's issues. They are not intended to be a straightjacket or to be asked of all persons. They suggest the kinds of questions and issues that pastoral caregivers will find helpful to listen for or ask about.

Spilka, Bernard, John A. Spangler, and Constance B. Nelson (1983). Spiritual support in life threatening illness. *Journal of Religion and Health*, 22(2) (Summer), pp. 98-104.

This study reports the results of conversations with clergypersons and with parents whose children died with cancer. The results about what parents perceived as being helpful and unhelpful are interesting. Overall, clergypersons reported a higher level of satisfaction with the care they provided than did the parents. That alone should make this article excellent reading for pastoral caregivers.

Stanton, Sarah (1994-1995). The use of art in pastoral care. *The Caregiver Journal*, 11(1), pp. 21-25.

This article is a very practical discussion of why and how to use creative expression as part of one's pastoral care. Although the setting in which the author developed this ministry is in the context of a hospital program, it is easy enough to translate into the ministry of persons based in congregations. The author makes clear how one can make use of a child's creativity without being a gifted artist one's self. Although this was published in a professional journal, libraries will generally be able to obtain a copy from an institutional library.

THEOLOGICAL REFLECTION

Allen, J. Timothy (1992). God talk and myth: Turning chaos into comfort. *The Journal of Pastoral Care*, 46(4), pp. 340-347.

This wonderful article explores how people use language about God during various pastoral encounters. The author draws parallels to the way ancient myths were used to communicate truths that everyday language was incapable of addressing. This article offers practical help to pastoral caregivers to reflect on what they are hearing and to respond in appropriate ways. Since children often lack the vocabulary to communicate what they are experiencing, the applicability to pediatric pastoral care is high. Although this is a professional journal, most libraries would be able to obtain a copy of the article upon request.

Culbertson, Philip L. and Arthur Bradford Shippee, Eds. (1990). *The Pastor.* Minneapolis, MN: Fortress Press.

The editors have culled readings from the patristic period to show what it means to be a pastor in the fullest sense of that word, both then and now. These collected readings and the commentary on them offer a wide variety of views. Potential readers should not be put off by the title. It is a very readable book by virtually anyone who is willing to read in small sections and think. Nor should readers be put off by the age of the writings. The problems facing humanity then and now are remarkably similar, and reading how early Christian writers faced them provides insights into contemporary pastoral care.

DeGruchy, John W. (1986). *Theology and Ministry in Context and Crisis.* Grand Rapids, MI: Eerdman's Publishing.

Written in South Africa, this book presents the concept of the minister in a congregation as the "theologian in residence." The book demonstrates how anyone can move from an experience to talking about it in terms of God. In the face of suffering, he argues how words about God must be spoken. There is a wonderful section on doing lay theology.

Weatherhead, Leslie D. (1944). *The Will of God.* Nashville, TN: Abingdon Press.

This book is based upon a series of sermons preached by the author to his congregation in London during the bombing of that city in World War II. He develops the idea of God having not one but several wills for humanity that exist on different levels. Although meant to address a particular evil, his answers also respond to anyone who asks the question "Why is this happening?" The book is easily read because the text was meant to be absorbed as a sermon and not an academic lecture; this is not to say that it is a superficial treatment of the topic. Although published in the United States, it is largely unknown, which is unfortunate because of its high quality and thoughtful approach.

Wolterstorff, Nicholas (1987). *Lament for a Son.* Grand Rapids, MI. Eerdman's Publishing.

This emotionally rich book is a father's account of his experiences after his son died while mountain climbing. It succeeds in speaking to the issues of why tragic events occur and how we might make sense of them because the author takes the reader along on his own journey for answers and meaning. This book would be an excellent gift for fathers whose children have died, particularly those who have died traumatically. Men who have difficulty expressing their feelings may find their voices through this author. The author wrestles with the issues of suffering and love in a way that makes this a theological book that is accessible to anyone.

Index

Order Your Own Copy of
This Important Book for Your Personal Library!

THE PASTORAL CARE OF CHILDREN

_____ in hardbound at $29.95 (ISBN: 0-7890-0604-9)

_____ in softbound at $14.95 (ISBN: 0-7890-0605-7)

COST OF BOOKS_____

OUTSIDE USA/CANADA/
MEXICO: ADD 20%_____

POSTAGE & HANDLING_____
(US: $3.00 for first book & $1.25
for each additional book)
Outside US: $4.75 for first book
& $1.75 for each additional book)

SUBTOTAL_____

IN CANADA: ADD 7% GST_____

STATE TAX_____
(NY, OH & MN residents, please
add appropriate local sales tax)

FINAL TOTAL_____
(If paying in Canadian funds,
convert using the current
exchange rate. UNESCO
coupons welcome.)

☐ **BILL ME LATER:** ($5 service charge will be added)
(Bill-me option is good on US/Canada/Mexico orders only;
not good to jobbers, wholesalers, or subscription agencies.)

☐ Check here if billing address is different from
shipping address and attach purchase order and
billing address information.

Signature_____

☐ **PAYMENT ENCLOSED:** $_____

☐ **PLEASE CHARGE TO MY CREDIT CARD.**

☐ Visa ☐ MasterCard ☐ AmEx ☐ Discover
☐ Diner's Club

Account # _____

Exp. Date _____

Signature _____

Prices in US dollars and subject to change without notice.

NAME _____

INSTITUTION _____

ADDRESS _____

CITY _____

STATE/ZIP _____

COUNTRY _____ COUNTY (NY residents only) _____

TEL _____ FAX _____

E-MAIL_____
May we use your e-mail address for confirmations and other types of information? ☐ Yes   ☐ No

Order From Your Local Bookstore or Directly From
The Haworth Press, Inc.
10 Alice Street, Binghamton, New York 13904-1580 • USA
TELEPHONE: 1-800-HAWORTH (1-800-429-6784) / Outside US/Canada: (607) 722-5857
FAX: 1-800-895-0582 / Outside US/Canada: (607) 772-6362
E-mail: getinfo@haworthpressinc.com
PLEASE PHOTOCOPY THIS FORM FOR YOUR PERSONAL USE.

BOF96